WEIGHT LOSS, LIFE GAIN

'A Motivational Journey to Permanent Weight Loss'

Chrissie Webber

Published by Accent Press Ltd - 2008

ISBN 9781906125813

Printed and bound in the UK

Cover design by Red Dot Design

**For my daughters
Ceri and Yvonne**

**With my love and thanks for all their care and
support**

ACKNOWLEDGEMENTS

I would like to start by thanking Christopher Ward for his help, support and enthusiasm. Most of all, I thank him for his constructive criticism, from which I learnt so much and this book benefited so greatly. He is a true friend, telling it as it is, holding back no punches and yet inspiring me to believe that I had a book worth publishing. For this, and his ongoing support and encouragement I will be forever grateful.

To my wonderful friend Anna Cherkas, I want to say thank you for teaching me what it is like to live as a person who has never dieted. She is the inspiration behind the habits of 'Conscious Eating'. Without her love and support in my life I would never have discovered what it is like to truly live without the fear of food, or the guilt and shame of eating it! Her ability to accept and love her body, its weight and size fluctuations between the seasons, inspired me to acknowledge what so many of us have discounted for decades – that every one of us is made uniquely different and very, very special.

Antoinette Glynn is another very special person. She touches my soul with her love and generosity. I thank her for that and all her work editing my book. Without her skill, wisdom and spiritual guidance in my life I would never have found the confidence in my writing or the nurturing spirit of love. This was the missing link within myself that finally inspired the messages in this book. My life is blessed because she is in it and because she has taught me so very much about happiness and unconditional love.

For his hard work, dedication, creativity and wonderful IT skills I must thank Andy Stroud. He took my concepts and made them visual as he created my web site *www.lifeshapers.co.uk* and my blog *www.chrissiewebber.co.uk* He probably doesn't realise this but with every new IT development, he inspired me to write in a way that would connect to my readers, as his visuals connected to me. It is through his skills that I am able to reach across the globe with my message that sustainable weight loss motivation is possible. For all of that, I am deeply grateful.

My love and thanks also go out to my dearest friend Jennie Gibbon – the sister of my soul. From the start, she read my chapters as they flowed off my computer. With each one she implemented changes in her life. She began her own journey to find the weight she was born to be and in the process became the motivation of my determination to touch as many people as possible with my writing. For all the times she is there to pick me up when the going gets tough; for all the love she shows me when mine is in short supply; for all the laughter she brings into my life and for a friendship that knows no bounds my thanks are eternal.

To Sandra Wynne who, with love and dedication to the concept of my book, edited my initial work. I thank her for pointing out to me how easily we take our friends for granted and how special that bond of friendship is when we nurture it with loving-kindness. Through our friendship she has inspired me with her creativity and fun. My book is enhanced by her thoughts and suggestions and my heart lifted by the friendship she gives.

Reaching across the globe to my dear friends Kerry Smith and Tril Schwerdt, I want to thank them for being my 'Body Image Enhancers' when I was in Australia. They made me remember the importance of dressing in what makes you feel a million dollars, not just sometimes but all the time. The fun days we spent together, as they acted as my image consultants, filled me with such love. I will treasure forever the time I had with them down under.

And finally to my daughters Ceri Hughes and Yvonne Webber, my love and thanks go out to them for the many ways they have taught me how precious it is to receive love. Their presence in my life was offered as a gift for my learning. They have taught me so much about myself and offered me a deep understanding of how special it is to love and be loved. There are no words that can express what they mean to me and so I simply thank them from the bottom of my heart

CONTENTS

INTRODUCTION

Let's get one thing straight from the start; this is not another diet book or quick fix eating plan. In fact it is nothing like the average diet or weight loss books. This is a book for people who are searching for a way out of the insanity of dieting. It is for those who believe that there has to be another way of living without shame, guilt, self-loathing or fear of food. That is, the 98% of people who want to lose weight permanently but never seem to attain their goal. These are the people for whom diets don't work as a long-term solution to weight, size and shape issues.

Within these pages you will unlock the secrets about why you have been trapped, probably for years, in an unhappy cycle of weight loss and weight gain. Its words bring to life the truth that sustainable motivation is the key to permanent weight loss. It highlights that, for most people, this cannot be achieved by a dieing mindset that is based on …

- Fear of food – 'good' food, 'bad' food';
- Fear of not being 'Good Enough';
- Fear of not being the 'right' shape or size.

This is because the key to sustainable weight loss motivation is not fear but self-love. As you read on you will discover what it is like to fall deeply in love with yourself. You will learn new habits of comfort loving that replace your comfort eating.

Each chapter takes you beyond the sets of 'can do', 'can't do' rules of the dieting game. They take you on a journey to reclaim the lost skills of 'Conscious Eating'. You learn how to stop your battle with food and regain your personal power. This is where you make your own choices about food and action through enabling your mind, body and spirit to work in harmony with food and nature.

As you delve into the pages you will find motivation in new and positive mindsets and beliefs. You will find a happier positive image of yourself and your body. The new beliefs can open up the truth, if you let them, to who you really are. Discovering the beautiful, radiant person buried within is part of the process.

Through this process you replace food with love as your comforter. Happiness is found here in life, a love of food, of self and the ability to fuel your body in a way that aids it in its search for the weight it was born to be. This where you find, at last, the motivation keys to sustainable weight loss.

HOW PASSION BECAME ACTION

I was angry and now I'm passionate. Angry that it took me decades to realise that the diets that had pre-occupied most of my life were never going to work. For me they were not a permanent weight loss solution. I was angry when I thought there was no way out of this battle with food, weight and size. Angry that I remained larger than nature intended, no matter what I tried to do about it.

All the diets, healthy eating plans, exercise and mental attitude training were to no avail. My motivation inevitably lapsed, at some stage, and the weight crept back on. As if that wasn't bad enough, I was also angry that all the messages surrounding me from the diet culture, made it clear that it was entirely my fault. And of course this reinforced my belief that I was not good enough. I was a failure!

The trouble with anger is that it's self-destructive. This negative emotion was not only eating away at me but also raising my stress levels and of course increasing my comfort eating. What a vicious circle I was in! I wanted to understand how I had got to this place – from an overweight child and teenager to a massive size 30 and over 21 stone by my mid forties. I wanted to find a way out of this misery. I wanted what everyone wants - to be happy. So I decided to turn the energy of my anger into a passion for answers and for a life of happiness and joy.

A PASSION FOR HAPPINESS

My passion for happiness and the truth grew as I began to realise that I was <u>NOT</u> a failure. Quite the reverse! The dieting mindset that kept me trapped as a victim to weight, size and food was failing me. Just think about it. How can you sustain motivation for permanent weight loss under a barrage of negative messages and beliefs?

How can a dieting 'Scarcity' mindset that makes food scarce and fearful by demonizing it – 'good' food, 'bad' food – sustain motivation? How can a combination of messages that reinforce that you are 'not good enough' if you are not a certain weight, shape or size, help you to lose weight permanently? How can obsessive focusing on food and weight aid in the motivation of weight loss? How can a negative body image make you want to love it, and look after it, even when you reach your target weight? All you have is a recipe for demotivation, NOT motivation.

That is unless you are amongst the 2% of people for whom this type of mindset works. The point is, we are all very different and so what works for one does not necessarily work for another.

The fact of the matter is, that for a majority of us, when food is made scarce in our lives we crave it more. Then, the more needy we are for it when it comes into our life again the more we reach out for it inappropriately. This is a quite normal reaction. It is a survival mechanism, as is our ability to store fat. In this part of the world, so abundant with food, most of us are never going to find happiness or the weight we were born to be – our body's set point – by making food our focus or our enemy.

By accepting the abundance of food in our lives and not fearing it, we are set free to develop a new and healthier relationship with it. This is an 'Abundant' mindset where the focus is on seeking happiness through life and not food. It is found through...

- A mindset of positive thoughts and beliefs (mind);
- Personal choice in determining the foods that fuel your body most effectively (body);
- Physical activity that keeps your energy high and your stress at bay (body);
- Self-loving actions that 'Feed Your Soul' (spirit).
- It works, not through placing your focus on food but on happiness and a joy of life.

FOOD FOR LIFE

For as long as I can remember, my life revolved around food. I grew up spending a majority of my time at home in the kitchen with my mother and sister. Food was used as a comforter, a reward and a social focus. Then in my teens I used it as a means of rebellion. In fact, I never learnt to have a healthy relationship with food, even in my formative years.

Eventually came my dieting years - over 35 of them! Through this period I learnt to fear food. I learnt to demonize it and to self-destruct on it. As I binged or starved, my level of self-loathing and guilt grew.

Like millions of others I learnt habits with food that kept me trapped in a daily battle with it. Mine was a spiral of depression and despair. Unhappiness, food obsession and weight gain saw my weight eventually spiral out of control.

Surrounded by messages that reinforced my belief that I lacked self-control, my self-loathing, guilt and comfort eating were perpetuated. I felt weak willed and simply 'not good enough'. A continuous battle raged within me and yet deep inside a tiny voice kept saying, "This is wrong, this is not the way life was meant to be."

Outwardly, in the presence of others I was full of life and fun, with an air of confidence in my over-sized self. Behind closed doors and in front of my family, a completely different person emerged. I was moody, angry, depressed, defensive, unlovable and deeply unhappy. I was larger than nature intended and I hated myself because of it.

Then the tiny little voice became more persistent; "It doesn't have to be like this, there is a way of losing weight permanently without all this angst and torment." So I began to reflect on the impact of the messages that bombarded my life. I thought about how they wrongly informed me that I was a failure and not good enough.

All this negativity was because of just one area of my life – being larger than nature intended. What about the rest of my life? Why did this one issue seem to trap me and hold me back?

Then I began to relate my situation to that of parenting. The more you tell a child they are bad or not good enough, the worse their behaviour becomes. Offering them little or no positive affirmations about how good and wonderful they are in many other ways only perpetuates their negative behaviour. The more you tell them they cannot have something, the more they want it and even demand it!

My dilemma with weight and food was no different. I was now the one parenting myself in a negative and destructive way. The whole pattern of my habits, beliefs and behaviour was set up wrongly. I was showing no understanding or love of myself. I was the one holding onto the negative thoughts, feelings and beliefs. I was the one beating myself up mentally most of the day. I was the one playing victim to life and food! It was time for me to take responsibility for my past, present and future thoughts, feelings and actions. The time had come to begin to change my life in ways that I never previously thought possible - to begin to really love myself.

So, the question I asked myself was "If I programmed myself to think and believe these negative things, could I re-programme myself for happiness, a joy for life and permanent weight loss?" The answer was YES! At last I had a life journey not a weight loss destination.

As I gradually unraveled the fears, thoughts, beliefs and habits that held me back from an abundance of love – love of food, of self, of life, of my body – my life changed. I reclaimed my personal power, taking charge of making choices that brought me happiness. I found happiness in new positive thoughts and feelings. I found happiness in the foods that made my body energetic and full of life. I found happiness in the self-loving actions that filled me with joy. I found happiness by focusing on living and loving life rather than loving and fearing food.

Finally, I found I was on a journey to discover the weight I was born to be. Don't ask me what that weight is, that's not the issue. There is no destination weight, just a journey of happiness. Have I lost weight? You bet I have – 5 dress sizes smaller and still slowly shrinking!

A JOURNEY

This book takes you along my journey. It is a journey of the choices I made. I offer it to you, not as a prescriptive plan of how to lose weight but as a collection of ideas, models and techniques. They are laid out here for you to choose from, as you create your own unique journey towards the weight you were born to be. Its first step is one of choice and an understanding that there are two doorways you can go through when times get tough or life is a struggle…

1   **The Easy Door** - This has a magnetic force that easily attracts you and propels you through. It is easy because you need do nothing to ease your journey through it. This is the doorway you go through when you are feeling…

- That there is no way out;
- Frustrated;
- Burdened and overwhelmed;
- Torn and dissatisfied;
- Hard done by;
- That others or society are to blame for your difficulties.

Although this is such an easy door to pass through, on the other side is dissatisfaction with life. Here the feeling of happiness eludes you. There is a lack of love and joy. The inner conflict and turmoil present you with a constant life struggle.

Then there is…

2   **The Secret Door** - This is the door that is sometimes hard to find. It is heavy to open, at first, because you are mostly pre-programmed as a human being to use the easy door. This is because the Secret Door requires you to…

- Accept 'What Is';
- Make an effort to use self-reflection and positive thoughts;
- Learn how to love yourself unconditionally;
- Observe and accept all the positive and loving things around you;

5

- Take responsibility for all your thoughts, feelings and actions;
- Examine and update your personal belief systems;
- Acknowledge, without blame, what you have done that has contributed to the difficulty you face;

or

- Accept, without blame, those things that happen to you through no fault of your own;
- Forgive yourself and others so that you can move on;
- Learn from this journey and stop repeating the old unhelpful patterns of thoughts and behaviours.

The effort it takes to move through the Secret Door really pays dividends. This is where you find your personal power. Here, you gradually find the person, shape, size and weight you were born to be. It is where true happiness, peace and joy live. With each small step in your learning and self-acceptance, you grow in self-belief, self-love and happiness.

What I first discovered within myself was a person I did not really know or like, and certainly did not love! I found that I had created in my life the loneliness and isolation I never wanted I had surrounded myself with people who treated me badly or didn't really want to spend time with me.

The truth is, I excluded them as much as they excluded me. I was a workaholic with no real time for my family and friends, except when I wanted them. Work was my purpose in life and food was my comforter. The 'Fat Jacket' (my excess weight) that grew around me to a massive 21 stone was my protection from what I saw as a hard, cruel world.

That was the world I had created, built on negative beliefs about myself. Within this world there was no room for love, not even for myself, although it was the one thing I craved more than anything else in life. Yet love always remained elusive. Why? Because I did not believe I deserved it! I never realised that to be loved, you have to first learn to love yourself.

I blamed everyone else for my unhappiness including the food I was eating. Never for one minute did I think that by looking within myself a new and joyful journey would begin to open up through the 'Secret Door'. It began to happen when I finally took full responsibility for inner, loving changes.

HOW TO MAKE THIS BOOK COUNT ON YOUR JOURNEY

This is your journey, if you decide to take it. The book is full of ideas, tools, actions and thought processes to effect change. These changes will replace a 'Scarcity' dieting mindset with a joyful 'Abundant' mindset. But this is your journey, not mine and so I have written the book to offer you choices for change. It is filled with the 'keys' to an 'Abundant' mindset. They form a treasure chest of choices for action. Take on board only those ideas and actions that fire your motivation. This book was not written as a plan that you should follow, but merely as a guide to inspire your motivation. Use the ideas as you see fit, adapt them and make them your own.

Your weight loss success is to be found through the ongoing positive actions you take that create the change and motivation you want. The point here is that inaction keeps you stuck in your old and unhelpful thoughts, feelings and behaviours. When you fill your life, every day, with new positive habits they eventually replace the old ones.

My words can only inspire. Motivation comes from within you alone. It is sparked from the inspiration you feel when reading certain words and ideas. Then it is enhanced by the actions you personally take to make the changes that are right for you. As a motivation coach, I know the best way for individual change to take place is for the person to commit to making decisions and taking actions for themselves. That is what I invite you to do as you read this book.

Make notes, mark the pages or sections where anything inspires or resonates with you. Just reading this book will not create change. Your motivation will soon wane if you don't take the actions that keep generating your ongoing motivation.

Better still - ask a friend who has issues with food, weight, size and shape, to join you as a 'motivation buddy'. Working together or in a small group is so much more fun. The support it offers can also be a powerful way to stay on track and keep your motivation levels high.

Having fun is not an option, it is a vital part of this process. After all, fun makes us joyful. That's exactly what you are trying to achieve through the development of an 'Abundant' mindset. So, this is where the fun begins and your battle with food and weight can end, if you want it to.

The focus of the book is on a love of life rather than a love of food. It is time to fall madly, truly, deeply in love with yourself, in a new chapter of your life. So, now I invite you to…

Learn to love life;

Learn to love yourself;

Learn to love food;

Learn to love change;

Learn to love happiness.

And in doing so I wish you…

A life well lived;

A body well loved;

A body image well cared for

And an abundance of happiness in discovering the person and weight you were born to be.

Chapter 1

Escape From 'Scarcity'

Over half the UK population is overweight or obese; in 2002, – 70% of men and 63% of women.

One in 5 adults is obese and obesity in children aged 2-4 years almost doubled from 5% to 9% between 1989 and 1998, in 6 to 15 year olds it trebled from 5% to 16% between 1990 and 2001

If current trends continue it is estimated that at least one third of adults, one fifth of boys and one third of girls will be obese by 2020!

CREATING A NEW MINDSET

Startling figures, yes! Yet it is thought that the only solution to the problem is dieting, or healthy eating. However, both of these can demonise many foods as 'bad', causing a 'Scarcity' mindset. In this mindset you create 'good' and 'bad' foods, making many of them scarce in your life. This in turn leads to an inevitable craving for what you want, but think you shouldn't have. The figures above clearly demonstrate that as a means of preventing or reducing the problems of long-term weight gain, diets and their 'Scarcity' mindset are not working!

If you want to lose weight permanently, a complete mind-shift is needed. A shift is needed that links mind, body and spirit in balance with food and nature. In other words, the 'Nurturing Spirit' of a loving 'Abundant' mindset. This is a mindset with an emphasis on self-love, which has at its heart…

- The healing of destructive thoughts and beliefs harboured about yourself (mind);
- A return to 'Conscious Eating' - the way food is viewed and used by people who have never dieted or had a weight or size issue (body);
- An increase in physical activity which has an emphasis on fun (body);

9

- An ability to tap into a nurturing energy, replacing food with love as your source of comfort, by 'Feeding Your Soul' with self-love, joy and peace (spirit).

Weight loss, through a balance of just mind and body, can of course be achieved. It happens when you get yourself in that 'right' frame of mind for dieting or healthy eating. You know the one; where you strictly follow the diet or healthy eating plan. Where you stick to the exercise schedule or the positive mental exercises. You just know that this time you will lose weight. And you do - for a time. Then it all goes down hill again! Pressure of work, emotions, relationships, feeling lonely and life problems eventually take their toll. They all impact on your stress levels and oops; there goes your will power and back come the comfort eating habits.

How familiar is that? So what's missing? The 'Nurturing Spirit' – a life force that replaces harmful thoughts, beliefs, messages and behaviour with self-loving actions and joy. Where does it start? It begins with the belief that you really are special, lovable and deserving of only the best. Where you see and are able to absorb all the love around you. Where you stop listening to what others say or watching what the media portray. And where you start listening to the 'Nurturing Spirit' within and around you.

Whatever you believe forms the reality of your life. When you focus on and see the negative, it clouds from view all the positive truths about you and your life. So if you believe yourself to be ugly, that's how you see yourself unless you believe ugly means...

Unique

Gifted

Lovable

Youthful

When you believe that you can't lose weight, your mind will easily be distracted away from positive thoughts and self-loving actions. It will easily slip back to the negative. These are the barriers that stand in the way of your permanent weight loss. Your actions are controlled by your thoughts and emotions. That you deserve to be happy and trim is without question. However, when you do not believe this you are doomed to reach out again and again, inappropriately for food. You believe the excuses you generate as to why you can't eat more healthily and take more exercise.

10

A positive inner self-belief is reinforced and held in place, like the cement in the foundations of a strong and beautiful house, by the power of love. This is the love you have always deserved. It is the love that eludes you in this area of your life. It is the love that is found in the very essence of the nurturing spirit. It is your love for yourself. It is the love that resides at the very core of who you are.

THE 'NURTURING SPIRIT'

At the heart of this love, within all of us, and within the world we live in is energy – a 'Nurturing Spirit'. When mind and body are in unison with this 'Nurturing Spirit' of love you find peace. Is that what you are searching for?

Peace of mind - positive thoughts about yourself;

Peace of body - wellbeing, energy and health;

Peace of spirit - the empty void filled with love and joy not food.

All around, the 'Nurturing Spirit' in the natural world creates harmony when we leave nature to run its own course. The power of this 'Nurturing Spirit' does not make everything perfect and regimented. It loves difference and diversity. It is only when we start to interfere with this diversity that imbalance and problems arise.

A dieting, 'Scarcity' mindset is one such interference. It throws our lives out of sync, mind and body out of balance with food and nature. Your mind no longer connects with what your body is telling you. This causes you to lose the ability to eat instinctively and know what and how much food your body really needs. You fill your head with negative and destructive thoughts - 'Not Good Enough', 'Shouldn't Have.' Negative and destructive emotions link with these thoughts – guilt, shame and self-loathing. These lead inevitably to negative and destructive actions. You eat food you don't need to find the happiness and comfort you crave. Most of all you block out the 'Nurturing Spirit' of self-love and give up on yourself.

When you love someone, you want only what is best for that person. You see the positive things in their make-up and character. You only want their happiness, joy and peace. Self-love means seeing the same positive aspects in yourself as you do in others. It is about creating loving action for yourself. After

11

all, how much do you show other people your love? What about yourself?

Without this self-love you struggle with the problems of your weight and size issues. So you struggle, not because you lack will power but because you lack 'Love Power.' That is, the ability to acknowledge and open yourself to an abundant source of love. Believing that you deserve and are 'Good Enough' to receive this 'Nurturing Spirit' of love, is the first step on a new journey through life.

The **'Nurturing Spirit'** of love is a sustainable self-love because it...

- Enables you to know at your deepest core that you are loveable and loved;

- Enables you to make positive connections with yourself and with others that reinforce how loveable you are;

- Strengthens your desire to know yourself in order to find the things that 'Feed Your Soul';

- Is accepting of yourself, just as you are;

- Enables you to share time, pleasures, thoughts and experiences that fill your life with joy;

- Gives positive support to you by allowing you to listen for what it is you really want, taking steps to make it happen;

- Enables you to find joy and peace;

- Fills your life with happiness when you choose to think and focus only on the positive;

- Enables you to know that you are capable of great things and allows you to open up your full potential.

If you are anything like me, when I first started out on my motivational journey to permanent weight loss, you will be thinking right now, "Well, I do love myself, so what on earth does she mean?" All I can say is that it's as if there is doorway to another level of love. Here is a level of love more amazing than you can ever imagine. Let me explain it like this…

When I was in the right frame of mind I would definitely love myself enough to eat the foods that filled me with positive energy and that suited my body (no indigestion). I would give myself the time to have lovely candlelight baths, a relaxing massage and time to exercise. The problem was, most of the time, I was doing it because I knew I should. Therefore, I was doing it not because I wanted to or because I found a deep joy in loving myself in this way. Sometimes I would even struggle, forcing myself to exercise or plan a weekend of activity for when I knew I would be alone.

Eventually when the positive frame of mind weakened, or when my life hit a crisis, the self-loving acts would drift away. This often happened before I gave up on eating the foods that suited me best. Because I did not truly believe I was worthy of all that love, my own self-love was not enough to sustain me through the ups and downs of life. All I wanted was someone to come into my life and give me love. The reality dawned; I was a fair weather friend to myself. That was just not good or loving enough!

A new year came and with it the realisation that no one else could make the changes to my life, only me. I began to realise that there was a greater power always available for me to tap into. The greater power of the 'Nurturing Spirit' was and always had been there for me to connect with. The only thing I needed was a positive mind to see it and an open heart ready to receive it.

Love is the very essence of the 'Nurturing Spirit', which provides you with…

- Inner Peace
- Personal Joy
- Self-fulfilment

Such are the results of an 'Abundant' mindset as you allow love to be your focus instead of food.

THE 'SCARCITY' MINDSET

However, the reality is that self-love has largely been forgotten. For nearly three decades we have allowed ourselves to be ruled by the dieting mindset. Its messages promote weight loss through dieting, with an emphasis on the perfect look, shape and size. All of this creates a constant struggle with life. This struggle raises your stress levels, increases your comfort eating and causes you to forget that you were born wonderfully unique. What also lies forgotten is the fact that your body knows instinctively what weight, size and shape it was born to be – it's body's 'Set Point'.

In this dieting, 'Scarcity' mindset you create a battle with food as the enemy. The battle is a daily one. It creates the emotional turmoil of wanting what you tell yourself you shouldn't have. Your emotions of shame, guilt, fear and self-loathing are out of kilter with those of love, joy, peace and happiness.

The more foods you make scarce by believing they are 'bad', the more you crave what you tell yourself you 'shouldn't' have. Your perspective on life becomes a battle of will. In battle there are seen to be winners and losers. In this battle most end up the loser!

Winners believe in themselves, they stand up for what they know is right for them. They listen to others but make up their own minds about what suits them. They define what it is they want and find their own way of achieving it. They see the positive even in adversity.

In reality there are very few winners in this dieting game when you believe that food is something to fear. In this mindset you will always be trapped in the illusion that being a certain size, shape or weight leads to happiness! Suppressing your winning and loving abilities, you 'play small'. You believe not in your true potential but in the false beliefs generated by this 'Scarcity' mindset...

- When I am a certain shape, size or weight, I will be happy and content;
- I lack will power if I am not able to lose weight and keep it off;
- If I am not on a diet or sticking to a healthy eating regime I am 'bad' and will put weight on;
- Foods are either 'good' or 'bad';
- I need to control my food intake by counting it, allocating points or colour schemes to it, if I am to lose weight permanently;
- Dieting by restricting 'bad' foods is the only way to lose weight;
- Fat people are lazy;
- Fat people are not self disciplined;
- Fat people are not loved or wanted.

14

Just surviving without gaining weight in this part of our planet, plentiful with food, can be a daily battle. It even becomes a daily battle where much of what we eat (or want to eat) is our dreaded enemy. The dieting propaganda perpetuates this culture of scarcity. Its focus is on all things external. There is a tendency to be controlled by what others think or expect. It instils in you the fear of food.

A belief that to be accepted as a valued member of society you need to conform to a desired look, shape and size predominates. Eventually you find yourself hooked into a life sentence! The weight loss market's billion-dollar industry is now so powerful that it has us believing that there is no alternative. Your constant fight with food and nature continues this belief, as you try more diets, fads or 'healthy' eating programmes. It simply is not true that there is no alternative!

The sad truth is that we have lost our ability to remember how to really love ourselves and to tap into the nurturing spirit. Fear of F.A.T. (Feeding on Anything Tasty) abounds in this culture the more that messages are distributed about the latest weight loss fad or diet regime.

Fed on stories of success, the diet culture blocks from view information about the sad truth. The truth that, for as many as 98% of people, diets do not work in the long term! For many they actually create weight problems for life and a diet dependency.

My journey to discover the weight I was born to be – my body's set point – began the day of my birth at a fragile 2lb 12oz. This saw me fight and struggle for existence! As the first born of twins I was exceptionally small and it was a miracle I survived those first few hours, let alone weeks. After some 3 months in hospital I was allowed home.

That was the start of me being 'fattened up'. You can imagine the pressure on my mother to feed me and make me strong. The timing of my birth also had an impact on my weight and size as I was born into post war Britain. Rationing had just been lifted, so the messages of eating everything on my plate resonate with me even today.

By the age of 18, I was a size 22 and to follow my chosen career in nursing I had to lose weight fast to be accepted on the nurses' training course. It was a dietician at the hospital who put me on the straight and narrow - a restrictive 1000 calorie a day diet. That was the beginning of my life of scarcity and dieting. I have lost track of how many diets and weight loss fads I have tried, over the past 35 years. Needless to say the only success I had was to lose weight and put it on again, plus a whole heap more! Sound familiar?

THE 'ABUNDANT' MINDSETS

By means of command and control the dieting 'Scarcity' mindset manages to take over your life. Escaping the insanity and regaining control over food by letting more love into your life, is easier than you may at first think. All it takes is a shift to an 'Abundant' mindset. This is a focus on self-love through inward reflection and personal choice. Its focus is on life, not food and the replacement of fear with the 'Nurturing Spirit' of love, peace and joy.

Left to its own ability, your body can naturally become and stay the shape, weight and size it was born to be. It can find its own 'Set Point', when you focus your life around the seven parts of an 'Abundant' mindset...

1   The Spirit of Love
2   The Spirit of Connection
3   The Spirit of 'Conscious Eating'
4   The Spirit of Time
5   The Spirit of Happiness
6   The Spirit of Healing
7   The Spirit of Activity

Within each part of the mindset are the lost pieces of knowledge that have been forgotten or obliterated by the 'Scarcity' mindset of the dieting game.

This process of changing mindsets creates a new and exciting journey. It takes thought and preparation. Yet for those who realise that there is more to life than struggling with food and size, the journey is one of great personal discovery and joy.

For over three decades my life was trapped in a quest for the right diet, the right frame of mind and the right exercise regime. Nothing ever worked consistently and for far too long I believed it was my fault.

The truth was I had been looking in the wrong direction for the complete solution to my weight, shape and size issues. I was on the right track, feeding my mind and body in healthy ways (at times). Yet, permanent weight loss still eluded me.

Then suddenly, I focused on the proof in my life that when the 'chips' were really down, a greater force than mine had always looked after me – the 'Nurturing Spirit'. I began to see that all the adversity I had faced in life, and overcome, demonstrated that I was already deeply loved and cared for. By holding love at bay, I not only created a food scarcity but a scarcity of everything in my life. At last I could see that this was a waste of good 'living time'.

With this realisation came a decision that life was too short to hide away in fear. It was time to stop filling my empty void with food instead of love. Waiting for things to happen that would make me happy was no longer an option. It was time to give up the struggle, stop playing the victim and make happiness my focus in life! So, I drew up a list of what I wanted more of in my life, that would increase my happiness...

- *A change in my mental attitude with a positive focus and far more appreciation of the things I have;*

- *A focus on the love and beauty around me and the self-love within me;*

- *A focus on being 'connected', in the moment, with my inner voice;*

- *A focus on a new and easy relationship with food;*

- *A focus on time to laugh; time to myself; time to spend with the people and on activities that fill my life with joy;*

- *A focus on developing my creative abilities;*

- *A focus on healing my body that I had abused through overeating and my mind through filling it with negative beliefs and thoughts;*

- *A focus on increasing the activity levels in my life to heighten my energy and motivation.*

The time had come to let go of any fears, focus on the joys in life and fully believe that I really deserved all the love and happiness I could find.

This is your personal quest, if you want it. A quest to find an alternative to dieting that still produces the weight loss or stability you have always dreamt of. The difference here is that there are NO quick fixes, only long-term gains!

17

The best things in life are those that take a little longer to achieve because they are sounder and more permanent. However, before you realise it the 'Nurturing Spirit' will be working through you. It will aid you in developing new ways of thinking and behaving. Soon you will be living a happier life where food is a friend and love is abundant.

Escape From 'Scarcity'

Top 10 Tips

1. Stop thinking of food as 'good' or 'bad'.

2. Choose to focus on all the signs in your life that point to the truth that you are beautiful, lovable and truly unique.

3. Look for your 'happiness fix' in life and not in food.

4. Believe that anything is possible, even permanent weight loss.

5. Stop listening to and believing the negative messages of the dieting mindset.

6. Remember, you will crave whatever you make 'scarce' in your life / mind.

7. Learn to love your body, even the wobbly bits!

8. Accept yourself, as you truly are – beautiful and lovable.

9. Stop trying to be what you think you 'should be' and find who you are without the food, weight, size and shape issues.

10. Stop believing that you're 'not good enough' and start finding the true depths of your inner beauty.

Actions To Escape 'Scarcity'

1 Feed Your Soul With...CHOICES FOR CHANGE with life and food.

Make a list of all the loving changes you want to make in your relationship with yourself and food. This is your 'Choices for Change' list. Really look at it and believe you deserve them. Commit to doing them for yourself. Take the lead where you want to share them with others. Ask the people you know and love to share their time, their love and their support with you on your journey. Build this list every day and start taking action.

2 Journey Log

Create a record by writing your own journey log. Buy a book to use as your journey log. Spend time looking for a really special one that is worthy of holding all your positive thoughts, feelings and actions. You may even want to buy a special pen to use or a set of coloured pens to make the writing come to life in colour.

Alternatively, buy a scrapbook and fill it with positive images of yourself, your journey and reflections of your loving mindset. If you are really creative try 'Scrap Booking' where each page tells a unique part of your journey and is elaborately decorated.

For those who like daily visual reminders of where you have been and where you are going on your journey, how about setting up a pin board. Put it in a visible place in your kitchen, study or office. Keep adding new pictures you have taken or cut out of magazines that represent the positive things that have kept your motivation high.

If you have a love of photography why not take lots of photos to represent your journey and put them up as new screen savers ever day/week/month.

At the start or end of each day, set aside just half an hour to create your log of the positive steps of your journey. Keep it private if you wish. Reflect back on it, especially when you hit one of life's inevitable problems. Reflect on all the actions you have taken to 'Feed Your Soul' each day. Note any ways you prevented yourself from reaching out for food. Note how you use the 'Nurturing Spirit' and note any positive changes in your beliefs, thoughts and feelings. Celebrate these (not with food!) and lift your motivation further.

When you write about or create a picture of what you have learnt, make sure it is coming from a positive perspective. If you do record anything that is negative make sure two or three positive statements or actions follow it.

As you reflect on your journey think about, and feel the joy of the self-love you are nurturing within you. Let this love spread to every cell of your body. Feel its resonance in your life and your world. Feel its glow and warmth within you and reflect on how you really do deserve it all, and much, much more!

Chapter 2

The Spirit Of Love
'Abundant' Mindset Part 1

For what is love itself, for the one we love best?
an enfolding of immeasurable cares which yet are better than
any joys outside our love

George Eliot

THE FEAR OF FAT

Love is at the opposite end of the spectrum to fear. Fear is like the threads of a silk cocoon. Each strand of fear is linked to another – fear of fat, fear of food, fear of not being loved, fear of not fitting in etc. All this achieves is the creation of an outer shell that stops you projecting the beauty within. It stops you seeing the reality of your potential. It stops you seeing and radiating the true beauty of who you are. It stops you feeling the love and energy of the 'Nurturing Spirit' that flows within and around, every moment of every day.

The fear of all fears - fat! That word, in a world of a dieting 'Scarcity' mindset, which none may mention for fear of offending. For so many of us, this fear generates an even greater one - that of not being on a diet, ever again. How on earth would you survive, surrounded by all this food if you were not on a diet or at least contemplating one? The simple answer is, by loving yourself so much that it…

- Fills the empty void within you, reducing your desire to comfort eat;
- Reduces stress levels due to the peace and happiness you feel;
- Fills your life with a focus on loving and living life to the full.

The key to permanent weight loss is to make self-love your focus by tapping into your 'Nurturing Spirit'. Change your 'Scarcity' mindset. Replace it with a new set of self-loving rules and boundaries that you choose yourself. Make them ones that lead to the creation of a life of abundant love where fear no longer reigns.

FACING FEAR - DEVELOPING LOVE

The only thing we have to fear is fear itself
President Roosevelt

Facing your deepest fears and letting go of them is an essential part of you journey to living life in abundance. All fears are based on the premise of loss and scarcity. When you see the world from this perspective you completely block from view all the loving abundance that brings happiness and joy. You lose the ability to 'be in the moment' and tap into the wonders of the 'Nurturing Spirit'.

Fear, in its insidious way, envelops all those who are hooked on the dieting game. It is the fuel that binds you to your belief that one day you will 'crack it' and find a diet that works.

Like a vortex it pulls into its centre more and more fears. All you see is the negative, all you hear is the negative and all you believe is the negative. Like a blanket it smothers the flames of your motivation, desire and passion to be who you were born to be. Fear hides from you the very nurturing spirit of the love you crave. Ironically, love will always be illusive in your life if you focus on fear. Which holds sway in your life, fear or love?

Where there is fear there cannot be love in the same moment. Fear smothers love, whilst love heals fear. Love is the key that will help you step out of the insanity of dieting. Its strength is undeniable!

When you allow your inner self to be consumed with fear, no love can get in or out. You behave in ways that make love and joy scarce. Your fearful behaviour pushes others away. It creates victims and losers. Love and its 'Nurturing Spirit' dispel negative thoughts and actions. It expands your world and connects you with everything and everyone in it. Love draws on the 'Nurturing Spirit' and attracts its positive energy to you. It is your choice – love or fear. Your challenge, if you choose to take it, is to replace the fears in your life with love. Love is an energy that brings with it great joy.

Claire suddenly interrupted my flow, as I talked about the nurturing spirit of love, by exclaiming, "Wait a minute, are you saying that whilst I am so busy working myself to a frazzle to make others happy and show them how much I love them, that I am missing out on seeing their love?

23

From my perspective it's that they rarely give love back!"

"Almost, but not exactly," I continued. "Sometimes we are looking in the wrong places for love. We often expect to see it in the format we are looking for, yet it is sometimes there in a completely different guise. For example, I always wanted my father to stop working and spend time with me. I wanted him to play with me, involve me in his world, hug me and tell me how much he loved me. I looked for years for these signs of his love and never found them.

Then I began to open my heart as well as my eyes and look for other ways he showed me how deeply he cares for me. There were dozens of them. Not only was I amazed, I stopped focusing on the negative – the things I wanted but never got. I began to focus on the positive and found the close loving relationship with him, I had always wanted." As Claire absorbed the information, I could see from the expression on her face that she had made the connection.

The result of a 'Scarcity' mindset is craving for all the things you believe you cannot have. It also leads to a neediness for all the things you fear losing. When what you believe is scarce becomes available again, you take too much of it in case it becomes scarce again. Or you hold on too tightly to that which you fear losing, only to lose it anyway as it dies within your grasp.

These patterns of behaviour come from a deep subconscious level, of which we are almost completely unaware. They are also motivation disablers. Once we realise what we are doing by noticing the times when loss, fear and scarcity underlie our behaviour, we have created an opportunity to make choices for change.

For much of your life you may have sought outward solutions to your struggle with food and weight. Now is the time to turn things around, looking inwardly to discover the causes of your fears, making new choices for change to break free from them. These are choices you make yourself in order to find your motivation enablers.

So, if that's the case, let me ask you these questions, "What's holding you back? What are your motivation disablers?" Is it the fear of giving up the controls and stopping dieting or the potential weight loss itself? Think about the answers you would give to this question…

IF I LOST WEIGHT WHAT WOULD HAPPEN?

Some possibilities are that you may…

- Attract attention from someone who wants a friendship/relationship;

- Lose your spouse/partner as he/she likes you to be big;

- Lose the love of a sibling/friend as she/he would be very jealous;

- Be without your protective 'Fat Jacket', so others see the real you;

- Be seen by others as weak and not strong;

- Be susceptible to illness if you were not big and strong;

- Not know who you are or how to act as a slim person;

- Not be able to be your usual extrovert and fun self.

By acknowledging your fears you have the choice to let them go. Do this by talking about them, writing them down, creating new and positive beliefs to replace the fearful ones. By facing the fear and doing it anyway you start a process of self-loving action.

Sadly, however, many of us learn techniques that block out the fear of ill health and the sustained unhappiness that accompany our weight and food issues. Yet, at the same time, there are many fears that are not locked in our subconscious. These also hold us back from living life to the full. These fears act against our potential weight loss. For example, they may be the fears of…

- Attracting attention to yourself…
  for fear of what others may be thinking/saying about your size.

- Having a go at something new and challenging…
  for fear of looking a big fat fool.

- Going out socially…

for fear of looking awkward, different and out of place.

- Going shopping for new clothes
  for fear of them not fitting or looking good on you.

- Letting someone get close to you
  for fear of them seeing the inner person you hate or are ashamed of.

- Having a great time by letting your guard down
  for fear that people will not like you.

Possibly the biggest fear of all, especially if you have spent a lot of time on and off diets, is the fear of giving up diets completely! Don't forget, this is a journey of personal choices. That means, if you want to keep dieting whilst undertaking your journey, that's just fine too.

"So what's the catch? I thought this was about getting off the dieting cycle?" There is no catch, just reality. As your journey progresses, so new skills with food grow and your focus changes. Gradually you find that food is no longer the issue. You are eating in a balanced and healthy way and enjoying life to the full. And so dieting is no longer the focus.

THE IMPACT OF OTHER PEOPLE'S FEARS

The fears of others, including your close friends and family can also be an obstacle on your journey. It is important to help them overcome their fears. The last thing you want is for them to influence you back into 'The Pit of Despair' - your old negative habits with food. Otherwise you lose sight of your destination. And you allow the 'Not Good Enough' beliefs to take their toxic hold over you again.

Communication is the key, as well as acceptance of other people's fears. Use your journey log to record your actions. Encourage those who are fearful of the changes to talk about the issues with you. Time and understanding of each other's viewpoints is all part of the journey.

In the words of Nick Williams, author of 'The Work You Were Born To Do', "Fear is the dragon that stands at the doorway of your success". The dragons you face on this journey may be few or many but what they guard is precious. They guard the realisation of your dreams, desires and the weight you were born to be.

These fears are personal to you. They are the very reasons you stop yourself from making choices for change and, more importantly, actioning them. The fiercest of all the fears is the one that holds you back every time. This is the one that you may not even know is there, or even want to acknowledge to yourself. Others are often the influence behind our fear without us knowing it.

Without realising the reason behind my determination to stay fat and happy – well, that's what I thought I was – I lived a façade for years. Under the surface of a personal and professional veneer, and behind closed doors, was the person I hid from the world. From my mid forties I struggled to get moving in the morning, as my joints were stiff and sore. Just walking any distance on the flat made me breathless. I suffered bouts of deep depression that I hid from the world. As for interesting life experiences, I avoided them like the plague even though there were things I longed to be able to do.

So, why did I not feel the fear that those who loved me felt for my health and wellbeing? Surely, this was the strongest fear of all - the dragon I needed to face? The answer was that deep within me a fear far greater than the loss of my health, happiness, and potentially my life, lay hidden. This was the fear that held me back from the shape and size I was meant to be. This was the fear of all fears for me, the dragon at the doorway to my success.

The fear was that, if I lost weight, I would lose the love and attention of my identical twin sister. Deep down I knew of her fear and jealousy of my losing weight and being slimmer than her! It seems so strange now to think what a strong subconscious hold this had over me. My skewed reality was that to lose my twin was worse than death itself, for me.

I finally realised that I can never lose her love because it has always, and will always, be there. As it registered within me that our deep, loving connection through the nurturing spirit is never ending, I was able to let go of my fear and lose weight again. Finally unlocking this deepest of fears gave me the chance to face it and move on.

"What on earth does all this 'stuff' about fear, have to do with weight loss and finding my body's Set Point?" I hear you ask. The answer is quite simple. By focusing on your self-loving, 'Nurturing

Spirit' and overcoming your fears, your focus is taken away from food. It is placed, once more, right where it should be on knowing who you really are and what makes you happy. The happier you are the less you reach out inappropriately for food.

GETTING TO KNOW YOU

It is a sad state of affairs that we don't usually stop and give ourselves time to really get to know who we are. Maybe that is because we are frightened of not liking what we may find. On the other hand, many are hoping to be looked after by that special someone who can fill their lives with happiness. The problem is that we rarely find one person who makes us perfectly happy all the time. That reminds me of a tale I heard that goes something like this...

Once upon a time there was a caring and sensitive person who, no matter what they did, felt empty and lonely. They longed for a special friend who would look after them and love them the way that they tried to look after and love the people they spent their life caring for. Then one day they met a wise old man and decided to see if he could help them in their quest. "For years I have searched for a special friend who would fill my life with joy and happiness," said the caring person. "Along the way I have met many who I thought would fit the role but eventually things didn't turn out as I had hoped and I moved on."

"That is sad," said the wise old man. "To find this person you must first understand these four things..."
The Special Friend *you seek may take a lifetime to find and get to know;*
The Special Friend *knows no limits to the love they feel for you;*
The Special Friend *can teach you much about yourself;*
The Special Friend *requires a special journey to find them.*

So the caring person packed all their belongings and went in search of ***The Special Friend****. The journey was long and interesting and they met many people who enriched their life, but nowhere could they find* ***The Special Friend*** *they longed for. Eventually they found themselves in the company of the wise old man again. "It is good to see you," said the caring person. "I hope you have been well since last we met?" "Oh yes," replied the wise old man. "How has your quest for* ***The Special Friend*** *gone, have you found them yet?"*

"No, though my journey has been long and hard," bemoaned the caring person. "I don't think I shall ever find the person I seek." Then

the old man smiled and said *"**The Special Friend** you seek has much to offer you so never give up on your search, simply remember these things..."*

The Special Friend is still waiting to be found;

The Special Friend will be with you always, once you allow them into your life;

The Special Friend, if allowed, will always have your best interest at heart;

The Special Friend needs no travelling to find.

*Ah, thought the caring person, I am finally in the right place. This is where I will find **The Special Friend** I have sought for so long. The years passed as the caring person enjoyed a life with no more travelling, being at last amongst new friends. Yet, as good as the friends were they never quite matched up to **The Special Friend** the caring person longed for. Then one day the old wise man returned to the village again and asked the caring person if they had succeeded in their search. "Since I stopped rushing around on my journey to find **The Special Friend** I have had time to really get to know people and have found such wonderful friends here but **The Special Friend** still eludes me," explained the caring person.*

*"That is such a pity. You have come so far and are so close to finding **The Special Friend**," explained the wise old man. "Let me offer you these thoughts one last time..."*

The Special Friend will always love you unconditionally;

The Special Friend will always fulfil your wants & needs;

The Special Friend is always there to lift you up when you feel down;

The Special Friend is always ready to listen to you if you open up a dialogue.

*The caring person sat quietly next to the wise old man, thinking deeply about the abundance of love and friendship that was to be found in life. As the caring person continued to relax and switch off their mind to the usual negative nattering that filled it, they began to think of all the wonderful things that had brought them joy over the past few years. Gradually they began to realise that as they stopped struggling with life, they had started to give themselves time and permission to pamper themselves and do some of the things that they had always wanted **The Special Friend** to do for them. Now they turned to the wise old man and began to tell him of other special things they had wanted to put in their life and how they were no longer going to wait to find **The Special Friend**. The wise old man smiled to himself for he knew that the caring person had at last succeeded in their quest and found...*

The Special Friend...
Was THEM!

What better friend could you ever want! You know exactly what it is that makes you happy. You know deep down exactly how to create joy in your life. You know exactly what you want to do and who you want in your life. All you have to do is listen carefully to your inner best friend without letting fear get in your way.

Then of course you have to take time to talk to and get to know your special friend. This may not be easy, given that fear is ever vigilant. It is through the power of fear that you experience your greatest sabotage to becoming the person and size you were born to be.

Fear and negativity are always getting in the way of you having a positive conversation with your inner best friend. They prevent you from taking action to bring peace and joy into your life. Fear really hates it when you get in touch with your special best friend as it completely diminishes its power over your life.

When you believe that there is abundance in all areas of your life, you love yourself unconditionally. You act in ways, which reflect the fact that you deserve all the love you can give yourself. That means creating balance in your life with some 'Me Time.' You look for and learn ways of keeping the fears and 'Scarcity' mindset out of your life. By doing this you replace the fears and scarcity with the only person who is with you from the cradle to the grave, to love and care for you...

YOU!

Yes, other people may come and go in your life, but if you do not love and care enough for yourself, then there is a scarcity. You are the main person who can add to the abundance of attention, love and care in your life. All it takes is time.

BEST FRIEND FOR LIFE

This is the start of you taking some 'Me Time'. Sit down and think about this very special friend. Imagine they are sitting right next to you now, what would you say to them? Remember, all new relationships start with a conversation. This may feel strange at first but as you get used to talking to your special friend, you realise just how great it is to have a friend whenever and wherever you need them.

Of course, your special best friend is not a substitute for other people. The remarkable thing is that, if allowed, they will encourage you to overcome your fears and expand your world of friends and experiences. Your inner friend can help you tap into your 'Nurturing Spirit' of self-love and set you free from 'Scarcity'.

Think about what encouragement you would like from your special friend. If you believe that anything is possible, what would you ask them for? This special person is found in you. There is an abundance of joy and love to be found in this new relationship. All you have to do is begin the dialogue. The rest is then up to both of you!

When I first discovered my very best friend, I wondered what on earth I would talk to her about. Once I started though, there was no holding back. We share...

- *Beautiful moments in nature;*
- *A quiet chuckle about situations I experience;*
- *Wonderful experiences on holiday;*
- *Sad times when I needed a shoulder to cry on;*
- *New ideas and inspiration;*
- *Feelings of uncertainty and doubt where I ask her advice and she gives me her expert guidance if I remove my fears and really listen;*
- *Situations where things need to be seen from a different perspective;*
- *Angry moments when I want to let my thoughts and feelings out;*
- *Times that I just want to be listened to without judgement;*
- *Doubts and uncertainties where I asked for positive alternatives;*
- *Discussions about what food I want to eat.*

FRIENDSHIP DATES

Life is too short and too precious to waste. So sometimes you need to spend time alone with yourself, on a 'Friendship Date'. These are the times you can focus more deeply on the joy of the moment. They offer you opportunities to 'Feed Your Soul'. These are the loving actions you take each day that lift your spirits. The experiences, places and events that make your heart soar with love and gratitude. They are the loving experiences created by you, just for you.

The problem is if you hate doing things alone, or you never enjoy them, you are not 'Feeding Your Soul'. Under these

31

circumstances you may have avoided doing things alone. You may have filled your time with negative thoughts of the past or fears of the future, failing to tap into the 'Nurturing Spirit' of the moment.

This is why taking yourself on a 'Friendship Date' is so important. These are special events you plan and get dressed up for. Putting fear and negativity to one side, you go out and experience the occasion with a focus on enjoying every moment. A 'Friendship Date', however, is in addition to time spent sharing the moment with family and friends, not instead of!

'Feeding Your Soul' is always enhanced when creativity, fun and play are part of the experience. Creativity heightens the moment, be it with or without someone to share it. This is because you open yourself up to the most powerful channel of the 'Nurturing Spirit' when you bring out your creative inner child. Consider how you can bring this fun and creativity into your 'Friendship Dates'.

To begin with, a 'Friendship Date' once a week is not out of line. If it builds your confidence to do things alone, lifts your spirits, and fills you with joy it is working. Once you have broken new ground and gone out on a date you will be longing to repeat the experience, if you have tapped into the 'Nurturing Spirit' of the moment. Planning your Date is part of the fun. Search the papers or Internet for ideas. Try the theatre, cinema, cultural exhibition, museum, art gallery, local events - the list is endless once you start the process.

- Don't wait to experience things in life you've always wanted to do.
- Don't play the victim and use your weight and size as an excuse.
- Don't allow yourself to get into patterns of negative thinking that spoil your date.
- Don't waste your time worrying what others may see, think or say.

Just remember, they are more than likely to be busily tied up in their own negative thinking to even notice you! And if they do stop and stare or pass comment, just remember you have the power of the 'Nurturing Spirit' on your side. Then consider how they have missed an opportunity of connecting in a positive way

to a very special person...
YOU!

The Spirit Of Love

Top 10 Tips

1.   Start to love yourself more than you ever thought possible.

2.   Remember that love is expressed in the actions you take to care for yourself.

3.   Face your fear – the one that holds you back from finding the weight you were born to be.

4.   Understand other people's fears and jealousies and don't let them influence you to give up on loving yourself.

5.   Replace comfort eating with comfort loving.

6.   Get to know and fall in love with yourself.

7.   Make sure you fulfil a self-loving act every day.

8.   Find that special friend within you and allow yourself to be loved – you deserve it.

9.   Go on a Friendship Date every week.

10.   'Feed Your Soul' not your face.

Actions To Fill Your Life With Love

1 Feed Your Soul With…your **Special Friendship Dates**!

Now it is time to plan and start going on your weekly 'Friendship Dates'. Trust me you will love it as long as you stop yourself getting into patterns of negative thinking. If you chicken out and stand yourself up for a date, don't worry, it is all part of the process. Arrange to do it another time and keep rescheduling until you do it.

Share your ideas and plans with a friend who is encouraging and supportive. It's also really great to share your experience afterwards with someone you trust. That way you relive the positive experience and feel the joy and elation all over again. By gaining encouraging support from others, your negative patterns of thought will not as easily make an impromptu appearance!

2 Journey Log

Write a brief account of your 'Friendship Date' and how you are celebrating your success (not with food!). This celebration is a very important part of your journey. Continue to keep a daily record of the positive actions you take as you focus on living life to the full. Make particular note of any changes happening in your eating patterns. Note the changes you make in 'Feeding Your Soul' instead of feeding your face!

You may even find it useful to make a list of all the things that would 'Feed Your Soul'. Use this list to formulate ideas for your 'Friendship Dates' and self-loving actions. These are the things that give you the 'feel good factor', for example…

- Taking a walk in nature in an area you would love to explore;
- Viewing a particular painting that inspires you;
- Creating a special sanctuary or loving environment for yourself.

Chapter 3

The Spirit Of Connection
Abundant Mindset Part 2

Ordinary riches can be stolen, real riches cannot.
In your soul are infinitely precious things
that cannot be taken from you.

Oscar Wilde

THE LOVING ACT OF CONNECTION

One of the first loving acts that requires attention after years of playing the dieting game is that of connecting back in touch with yourself and life. For years you may have only been connected to food. Your focus may have been on wanting it, thinking about it and allowing it to rule your life. This focus may have obliterated the loving connections in life that bring happiness and joy.

So on your journey through life are you connected or disconnected? When you live your life in an 'Abundant' mindset...

- your mind is connected to the feelings of your body;
- your mind is connected to your fuel tank – your empty/full feelings - to ensure that excess food is not wasted (put on our waists and hips!);
- your mind connects to life in the moment – the power of the present;
- your mind is connected to your inner friend and the loving things that 'Feed Your Soul';
- your mind is connected with the energy that each food provides in order to determine those that are the best fuel for your body;
- you are connected with your own inner beauty;
- you are connected to your deep intuition;
- you are connected to your emotions and thoughts and so avoid comfort eating.

Through this mindset you fully connect with the abundance of joy and beauty in the world around you. You connect with the positive things people say, not the negative ones. You are healthily connected with the food you eat. In this mindset you seek, and find, the abundant connections with the joy and happiness you deeply crave. The disturbing thing is, when you are disconnected, you think you will find happiness at a certain weight, size or shape. This is the illusion that a 'Scarcity' mindset creates!

MAKING CONNECTIONS
Through our unhealthy connection with food we allow ourselves to be influenced by outside forces. When we spend a long time in a 'Scarcity' mindset we switch off our mind-to-body connection. In doing this we ignore the messages our body is sending us. We switch off our connection with our inner emotions and stresses by burying them with food. We eat without any consciousness of our body's feelings.

Even when we are vaguely aware of being over-full, we still manage to stuff in that extra dessert! On the other hand we may even ignore the hunger pangs as we starve ourselves to lose weight. How sensible is that?

Having lost touch with the connection to our body and its feelings our connections are transferred to all things external. In other words we focus our attention on our food, size, shape and weight. We therefore, make connections that so often reinforce in us that we are 'Not Good Enough'...

- Some of the food we eat is seen as 'bad';
- We think critically about how we look;
- We look at others and compare them with ourselves;
- We listen to the negative things others say about us;
- We fill our minds with our perception of what others think about us.

What nonsense we then generate within! Never connecting to the 'Nurturing Spirit' through our inner, loving self we lose touch with the person we really are. We struggle to become the person we think we should be – the one that fits the dieting game profile. What is lost, in this process, is the skill of connectedness with the person we were born to be. This is the skill of linking mind, body and spirit in harmony with food and nature.

For a long time I thought I had overcome the power of the dieting mindset by connecting back with myself. Later, I found that this was the wrong form of connection. It was a negative, destructive one that said, "Blow this dieting. I am who I am." I had given up my battle with food to be able to wear my 'Fat Jacket' (my outer shell of excess weight) and be happy.

How wrong could I be! This was not happiness, as I now know it. However, at that time all my friends were of the same mindset. My desire was so great to 'fit in' that I surrounded myself with like-minded people - my 'Me-too-Gang'. These were the people I could rely on not to comment about what, or how much, I was eating. This was the gang who believed that dieting was a waste of time. They believed being fat was not a problem. After all, the research into health risks was a load of rubbish, wasn't it?

I realise, that in my particular 'Me-too-Gang,' there was a very destructive member, known to me as 'Pro'. He was the person who kept me from eating sensibly - the Procrastinator to give him his full title. For a long time he was my life-long buddy. When the toxic 'Not Good Enough' beliefs managed to break down my usually impervious resolve to be fat and happy, 'Pro' would always be there. His role was to generate the most compelling reasons why I would not be able to start a diet or take some exercise just yet. He was always so convincing when he filled my thoughts with suggestions such as...

- *It's not Monday and everyone knows that's the best day to start a diet!*
- *That shoulder injury might return if you went swimming regularly again;*
- *All the fresh fruit and vegetables you buy will only go mouldy and be wasted as usual;*
- *There is still that chocolate in the cupboard, so no use starting a diet until the temptation is out of the way;*
- *You're going out to dinner this week so leave it until that's over.*

There were also people who tried, at every possible occasion, to make me feel guilty or frightened – or so I thought. These were my 'Rescuers', the people who because they loved me, felt it their duty to help me out of my 'Fat Jacket'. They seemed to regularly point out what I was doing wrong. Many times they would tell me what I should be eating or the newest diets they had read about.

Oh boy, that's all I needed, people pointing out that I was doing it all wrong. I felt so persecuted when that happened. My store of 'Not Good Enough' beliefs would be full to overflowing by the time they were finished. That would make me really angry. Often I would retaliate by going on the attack. Worse still, I would become defensive and then end up feeling like the victim. My belief that I was different was heightened to a point of painfulness. I thought myself weak-willed, lazy and just stupid not to be able to lose weight permanently. And where did that all lead? To more inappropriate comfort eating of course!

I even developed a number of subconscious tactics to keep the 'Rescuers' and their negativity at bay. One tactic was to throw an emotional 'wobbly' when confronted by their messages or comments. This was often successful at keeping them away for long periods of time. Another tactic I used was to completely ignore whatever they said. Of course when the occasional message did creep through I always had 'Pro'. In addition I had my 'Me-too-Gang' to turn to for support and reinforcement that whatever the 'Rescuers' said should be ignored.

Therefore I firstly, connected myself to food. Secondly I connected with a few people who were either like minded or knew better than to point out that I was unhealthy and unhappy. In my mind they had to love me for who I was, not what I looked like. It never occurred to me that they loved me enough to be worried about my health and happiness.

Food was my friend and my comforter. I would connect with it in times of stress or emotional turmoil. When I felt empty and alone, food would be there to make me happy by burying my emotions. Scathing in my attack against dieting, I was determined to be fat and happy rather than have to give up the wonderful foods I loved – well, thought I loved! What other alternative did I have?

The truth of the matter is that there are alternatives. When you learn to connect, in a positive way, with more than just food, life changes. This is the process of connecting with the 'Nurturing Spirit' of love within you. Even if you are already pretty good at giving and receiving love, you will be surprised how much more there is. You will be amazed at what you have been missing, once you connect with your inner self.

CONNECTING MIND TO BODY
Connecting your mind to your body is a vital action to take as you relearn the skills of an 'Abundant' mindset. Years of ignoring what your body is telling you will have taken their toll. The types and amounts of food you eat, their effect on your body and the way you think about food needs to change. Connecting mind to body allows you to identify…
- food satisfaction levels;
- emotions that cause your comfort eating;
- types of foods that have a detrimental effect on your body;
- types of food that give you the most positive energy;

- types of activity that raise your energy and motivation.

You learn to connect, once again, to your body and personal 'fuel tank'. Through these connections you discover that food is energy giving when selected to suit your unique body and eaten in the right proportions. Even the foods that do not suit your body will be perfect for another person. As you begin to eat and live for energy and joy, you become re-connected to your power of choice. By making no food 'bad', it loses its power over you and craving becomes a thing of the past.

If you are allergic to certain foods or a certain food, and they have a detrimental effect on your body (e.g. sugar for diabetics), it does not make the food 'bad'. It just means that for you it is an ineffective fuel source. Accepting 'What Is'- the reality of your specific food needs - is important. Finding alternative foods that you enjoy as much, if not more, is the key to not feeling deprived. Once you dispel the feelings and thoughts of certain foods being 'scarce' in your life, the cravings stop.

Another way to get rid of these cravings is to know that you can have the food at any time you want. The key here is one of thoughtful choice. This is where you carefully consider the effect the food will have on your mind and body. You then consider choosing alternative foods you will enjoy just as much, if not more.

Within this mind and body connection lie the forgotten habits of 'Conscious Eating'. These are the habits of people who have never dieted. Learning or re-learning the skills of 'Conscious Eating' is one of the major keys to living in a world of food abundance. You will read more about them in the next chapter.

CONNECTING WITH LIFE IN THE MOMENT
The longer you are trapped by the 'Scarcity' mindset of dieting, the more your psyche gets used to the pain of your negative emotions. In a strange way you may even form a perverse relationship with the pain and negativity. This happens when you are strongly connected to identifying yourself as a person who struggles with weight and size. It is fuelled by your ability to absorb and believe the things that highlight and reinforce that you are 'Not Good Enough'. Its outcome is that you fail to connect with the present moment and enjoy life to the full. You miss seeing an abundance of evidence that shows the reality that, no matter what has gone before, you actually are 'Good Enough'.

40

Take a moment to think about your negative thoughts and emotions, the ones that…

- Constantly reaffirm that you are 'Not Good Enough';
- Rear their ugly head as a starting point to your comfort eating;
- Increase as you withdraw from problems in your life.

Every single one of these thoughts and emotions is filled with negative energy. This energy comes from one of two places, the destructive memories of the past or the fears of the future.

These memories and fears keep you trapped, fluctuating between two states. You play victim to your own thoughts and emotions when you fail to use the power of the present moment.

I had forgotten what it was like to live guilt-free, without fear of food or struggling with my weight, shape and size. Exposed to "Not Good Enough" beliefs since birth, I developed a protective layer around who I was born to be. This was my 'Fat Jacket' - my excess weight.

Some of my friends reached their teens or adulthood before their exposure to 'Not Good Enough' beliefs caused them a problem. It propelled them into a life of dieting. All our situations led to the development of this protective layer around us - our 'Fat Jackets'. Just like flak jackets, worn as protection in battle, we developed them to protect our vulnerable inner self. It formed a protection against the ravages of the 'Not Good Enough' beliefs – our own and others'. Aided by our own fears, and the negative influences of the continuous distribution of media messages, our warped sense of reality was sustained.

The negative influences that escalate 'Not Good Enough' beliefs come in many guises. One such guise is 'airbrushed' photos that make people appear far thinner than they really are. Their influence has us aspiring to be the shape and size of models. I realised how insidious this was when I discovered that most models weigh as much as 23% below the normal body weight thresholds. This puts them into the percentile range of those with eating disorders!

Gradually I became aware of the long-term effects of exposure to the power of the "Not Good Enough" beliefs. For a long time I was convinced that dieting and a 'Scarcity' mindset was the only way to lose weight. At times my fear of my weight issue became so strong that I adopted an avoidance mindset. My personal health and wellbeing was ignored. Trying to escape I only found the same problems, though cleverly disguised, in the latest healthy eating ideas. Here, food was still identified as 'good' and 'bad'. I remained unaware of the powerful 'Nurturing Spirit' that had always been available to me in the power of the present moment.

Once hooked into a pattern of dieting, my problem was that within a two to five year period any weight loss was regained. Frustrated and unhappy I put the weight back on, plus at least an additional 10%. Because of this, I would eventually return to long periods of R & R - Repetitive-Eating and Restful-Recuperation. This was a life without dieting, in an 'Avoidance' mindset, where weight gain was still an issue. Then I had periods where I fluctuated between an 'Avoidance' mindset and a 'Scarcity' mindset - yo-yo dieting. My life was full of despair and unhappiness. My behaviours, especially when I was yo-yo dieting, were not normal. They were unhealthy at best and obsessional at worst!

The sad thing was, for some of my friends who dieted like myself, there had never been a need for them to diet in the first place. They had not been overweight to begin with. They just thought they were. The 'Not Good Enough' beliefs, generated by the diet culture, had worked their dark magic. The longed-for permanent weight loss, which they never originally needed, became long-term weight gain – a life sentence!

Some of my friends who did lose the pounds and keep to their target weight still struggled obsessively with food. Their continued 'Scarcity' mindset had a negative effect. Life for all of us was a constant cycle of food restriction and exercise obsession. The daily intake of 'Not Good Enough' beliefs was so high that it created a struggle with life, bringing with it pain and demotivation. Beneath the veneer of contentment, inner peace, joy and happiness were almost unknown. Many of us seemed happy enough because, at the time, we had no idea that all around us, and deep within, there was a 'Nurturing Spirit'. It was here that another level of joy was blocked by fear of food, weight and size.

As much as we want to rid ourselves of this problematic repetitive behaviour, we keep revolving back to painful thoughts and emotions. This is because they are more familiar to us than the joyful ones we long for. It is therefore not a problem that can be solved by dieting or by positive mental attitude techniques alone. What is missing is the third and vital dimension of a life of abundance – the nurturing spirit of love found in the moment. This is where 'The Power of the Present' resides.

You are given 'Now', to connect with its beauty, energy and joy. The happiness it offers is a powerful healer and an uplifting

'Nurturing Spirit'. It is the present moment you are given to use as you wish. The choice is yours…

- You can waste it by not noticing it;
- You can waste it by filling it with negative thoughts or emotions;
- You can waste it by being focused on a negative mindset;
- You can waste it with fears of the future;

OR

You can use it to top up your happiness reservoir, whenever you want.

For many of us the past and the future are painful or scary places on which to focus. Yet we still spend most of our daily life in one or other of these mental arenas. We may try to focus on the positive, remembering positive events of the past or projecting positive mental images of the future. However, it can be a constant struggle as you try to focus on the positive. The reality is that all your mind wants is to concentrate on the negative.

With practice I became fairly good at focusing on the positive. I would spend time every day chanting affirmative statements and creating positive visualisations in my head. I would see myself as a size 12, wearing a slinky black evening dress. Eventually though, my focus would shift back to the negative influenced by some external event. That would bring my carefully constructed pack of positive cards tumbling down again. I would be back in my negative thinking.

My 'Not Good Enough' beliefs would flood back to the surface. My mind would be back in 'Scarcity' mode. Again I would find myself believing that not only was I a failure at dieting, I couldn't even master the mental techniques of positive thinking.

What I eventually realised was that when we focus negatively on the past or the future, we miss out on the very place that joy and the 'Nurturing Spirit' reign - the present moment. This is where we are able to find joy, unhindered by the pain of the past or fear of the future. The present moment is so powerful because…

Yesterday is history,

Tomorrow is a mystery,

But today is a gift – **The Present**

The history of all your yesterdays can influence your future in a positive or negative way. Through your remembrances of only

43

the problems and negativity, you influence more pain and problems in your tomorrows – your future. The gift you have is in being able to stop and change the way you view the history of yesterday. It is within your power to positively influence the mystery of tomorrow. By refusing to allow yesterday's negativity to influence the joy, beauty and peace of the moment, you give yourself the present.

With our minds so full of negative chatter we fail to fully see and appreciate what we have that is wonderful and precious in life. Not only that, we fail to tap into the source of the 'Nurturing Spirit' found in the present moment. It is this source that can fill our empty void, bring us peace and offer us all the love we could ever wish to find. Just as we choose the actions we take every day, we can choose to bring more joy, peace and love into our lives.

Not convinced yet? Then bear with me and try out the 'Power of the Present' and see how much peace and joy it brings. Take a walk somewhere you like, a park, the countryside or your garden. Go alone and spend at least half an hour walking round. Begin by placing your focus on the beauty of the things around you. Slow right down, so that you take in the detail of a leaf, a flower, the bark of a tree. Stop and really study something that takes your interest.

Be like a child, inquisitive, noticing every intricate detail. Feel and smell whatever it is you are focused on. Open up all your senses of sound, touch, smell and even taste. Let go of any thoughts that come into your mind, especially the negative ones. Let go of worrying what others may think. Begin to feel the negative energy fall away as you tap into the positive 'Nurturing Spirit' of the moment. Don't fight with any thoughts that come into your head, just acknowledge them and let them go. Nothing else matters just the power of the moment. Feel within it the joy and peace that lift your spirit and 'Feed Your Soul'.

Now you have experienced the beauty and love in the moment, just think how much more comforting this is than eating. There are many more ways to tap into the power of the present that will unfold to you as you read on. It is one of the 'gifts' that you can give yourself, every day, to 'Feed Your Soul' instead of comfort eating.

CONNECTING WITH YOUR EMOTIONS AND THOUGHTS

When something is missing in our life, or when things get too tough, many of us fill the void with food. We comfort eat as a means of avoiding and burying the difficult issues that life throws at us. These include the painful emotions that accompany them. We turn to food as our comforter. Yet, no matter how much we focus and 'feed on food' it never solves our problems.

I sat alone on the sofa, the television droning monotonously in the background. The box of chocolates on my knee was almost empty. Tears flowed down my cheeks as I stuffed another chocolate in my mouth. I knew I was slowly killing myself. I felt trapped, weak-willed and unable to lose weight permanently. I had no connection with what I was feeling. I had no understanding of why I needed to stuff myself until I felt sick. I had no connection with what I was eating and no way out - or so I thought.

I was alone, disconnected from everyone and everything except food. Still I was unhappy. "I don't want to be alone," screamed in my head! And yet I had created my own aloneness. At last I began to realise that none of my problems had anything to do with food or size. They were all about how I disconnected myself from life and all its abundance. My soul was empty and crying out to be filled with love from myself. Then my exploration of the nurturing spirit began.

Each time you reach out for food as a comforter you are ignoring the fact that your body really wants loving comfort, not food. The problem for many of us is that we are connected more to food than we are to our emotions and ourselves!

Used as a stress reducer, a substitute for love and a means of burying our emotions, food only makes our weight issue worse. It solves nothing. It does not bring the joy and peace we crave. Instead it offers only momentary comfort followed by shame and guilt! Connecting with our emotions helps us to reduce the amount we comfort eat.

Food never really fills the void or gives you lasting comfort. How could it? Yet you hold tightly to the illusion of the comfort of food! This belief leads you into a spiralling decline until all you see in your life is that food counts – calories, points, colours – you are hooked on dieting. We 'feed our faces' to fill the void. We feed our bodies whether the diets are working or not. Do you ever consider the importance of 'Feeding Our Soul'? Of loving yourself enough to open up to the nurturing spirit? 'Feeding Your Soul' with self-loving actions that make your heart sing and fill your life with joy replaces the food you do not need.

CONNECTING TO FEED YOUR SOUL

'Feeding Your Soul' takes a conscious effort as you search for joy and happiness instead of pain and shame. It means refusing to play victim to food, weight and size. It means refusing to bury the problems and emotions you face. It requires you to start searching for the things in life that give you 'the buzz'. These are the ones where you ...

- Get the 'wow' factor;
- Feel elated;
- Experience an event or the moment that fills you with joy;
- Laugh until you cry or cry because you are touched by loving words or deeds;
- Feel the love given freely to you from friends and family;
- Share the moment with family, friends or someone special;
- See something that takes your breath away;
- Experience the simple joy of a bird in flight or a morning shaft of sunlight touching the land;
- Spend time immersed in a hobby or in touch with your creativity;
- Give time to yourself for the simple pleasures in life;
- Are doing things alone that bring you happiness and joy.

These are just some of the things that can 'Feed Your Soul'. Like choices of food to feed your body these are choices of actions to 'Feed Your Soul' every day. Try as we may, we cannot replace the need to connect with our spirit of self-love. Starved of its presence in our life, nothing can ever substitute the nurturing spirit that 'Feeds Our Soul'. It offers a healing process that you will read more about later.

It is comfort-loving actions that 'Feed Your Soul' – filling you with happiness, joy and pleasure and reducing your comfort eating. Here are some unconditional acts of love that you can do for yourself...

- Bathing by candle light;
- Indulging your creativity;
- Treating yourself to a luxurious massage;

- Making new friends;
- Spending time pampering yourself.

As you 'Feed Your Soul' with your self-loving actions you overcome the stresses, fears and emotions that keep you locked in the habits of comfort eating. By focusing your attention on abundance and the wonderful choices it offers, life becomes more enjoyable. You make food your friend and not your enemy. Your cravings stop and weight loss is achieved with ease and joy.

Your goal is eating to live, not living to eat. The difference is subtle yet important. By investing so much time and attention on the food you eat, the best things in life can so easily pass you by. Eventually your relationship with food becomes more important than your relationship with yourself.

We have forgotten that eating is a process that fuels our body so that we can go out and enjoy life! When we eat for comfort we do it to avoid reality.

CONNECTING WITH THE REAL YOU

'Feeding Your Soul' is never going to help if your world is not based on reality. So how much of your life is spent disconnected from reality? Are you a proud owner of a 'Deception Mirror'? This was what I once owned. These are very exclusive and treasured possessions. They allow the owner to see a totally different picture of themselves. It has the power to warp perception and shows a reflection of the user that exaggerates all their negative traits.

On the other hand you may be one of those people who do not possess a mirror of any description. In fact, mirrors may be banned from your house in order that not even a glimpse of reality can be seen!

Wouldn't it be wonderful to live on a planet where there were lots of mirrors that all showed the truth about you – a reflection of your inner beauty? Actually, everyone has an inner beauty that radiates when you really know and love yourself. People who are heavily overdosed on the 'Not Good Enough' beliefs have a warped perception of who they are and what they look like. These 'Not Good Enough' beliefs', when generated and held in the mind, do not have your best interest at heart. So it's time to start believing that…

YOU WERE BORN BEAUTIFUL INSIDE AND OUT

Accepting ourselves as we are and acknowledging what we can and can't change is vital to our journey. Think about your family in terms of their shape and size as individuals. How would you describe your family traits - pear shaped, heavy set, short legs, round body? Take a look at those old family photos. Begin to build up a picture of the real genetic make-up you were born with.

Its no good trying to change what you were born to look like, in general body shape terms. This is a pathway to constant grief, so let's get real. No matter how much we diet or exercise most of us will never achieve that model look we hanker after.

Isn't it time to make the most of what we do have? Isn't it time to learn to accept and love ourselves as we really are? The greatest thing we can change is the way we see ourselves. We can change how we love and accept ourselves, no matter what our shape and size.

As you may already have realised, perception is not always reality. Your perception of the shape you want to be, if it does not fit with reality, will only cause you great stress and pain as you try to attain the unattainable.

Connecting to reality and learning to love every part of yourself unlocks the doorway to your inner beauty. This beauty then radiates for all to see. Even your 'wobbly bits' can be loved the more you connect with the 'Nurturing Spirit'. The reality is that the more we love ourselves, the more attractive we become because beauty is not skin deep, it is soul deep.

The Spirit Of Connection

Top 10 Tips

1. Perfect your ability to switch your mind onto your body.

2. Get in touch with your intuitive side and listen for the messages that tell you that you're on the right track.

3. Connect with your emotions and take action to accept them rather than bury them.

4. Connect with your inner beauty; feel it; believe in it; let it shine forth.

5. Be watchful of the ways you disconnect from yourself and your emotions before you comfort eat.

6. Connect to the moment and feel the joy of being free from past negativity and future fears.

7. Connect to the energy in the food you eat to determine the fuel that suits you best.

8. Connect with reality – stop battling against 'What Is', you will never win.

9. Connect to the beauty all around you in the world and the 'buzz' for life.

10. Connect to the 'winner' within you and give up the struggle that keeps you trapped as a victim to food.

Actions To Connect

1 Feeding Your Soul Through…a selection of **'Soul Full Moments'.**
How about making time each day for a number of 'Soul Full Moments'? Half the fun is in switching your total awareness to the moment. So think of ways of connecting with the present moment. Think of the activities that lift your spirits and could fill the void you usually fill with food…

1. Listening to the birdsong in a morning;
2. Singing or playing a musical instrument;
3. Watching for the loving moments between family and friends;
4. Feeling the breeze on your skin;
5. Smelling the newly cut grass.

Develop a toolkit of 50 actions which 'Feed Your Soul' –

- People
- Places
- Activities
- Events
- Self-pampering
- Exercise
- Creativity

– and reduce your comfort eating. Place a copy on the fridge door and then take action each time you want to turn to food. If it's stress or emotions that make you reach out for food, think about the triggers. Plan some 'Soul Full Moments' ahead of time to reduce the negative impact of your thoughts and feelings.

2 Journey Log
Fill your log with a list of the all the ways you want to start connecting with yourself and the world around you. Include positive responses that change your focus and help you connect with the 'Nurturing Spirit' of your inner, self-love. Consider the barriers you put in place that prevent you making these loving connections and list the actions you will take to overturn them.

Chapter 4

The Spirit Of 'Conscious Eating'
Abundant Mindset Part 3

*It is the food which you furnish to your mind
that determines the whole character of your life*
Emmet Fox

EAT CONSCIOUSLY

For many years you may have been disconnected from yourself, busily focusing on the dieting game. You may therefore have forgotten the skills of eating consciously with your mind fully connected to your body. This was something I learnt from a friend...

Some years ago I was on holiday with a friend who had never dieted in her life. As we sat in the hotel restaurant some fellow guests stopped at our table to discuss the fantastic spread of food available to us at the buffet. On extolling the virtues of the dessert section they asked inquisitively, "Aren't you having one?" To our reply of "No, actually we're full", they retorted with the much used, "Aren't you being good!" My friend was amazed as, believe it or not, she had never in her life heard this much-used phrase.

What followed was the first of many interesting discussions. Its focus was on the differences in how food is viewed and used by dieters, as opposed to those who have never dieted. It was then that I began to realise the importance of the connection between my mind and my body. In listening to how she viewed and used food, so differently to myself, I began to learn the skills of 'Conscious Eating'.

So, what are the differences between those fortunate non-dieters who have never had a weight problem (real or perceived) and those of us who diet? Firstly, they see food in all its abundance as a source of fuel. This gives them an advantage over dieters. They have no reason to crave food, because they can have anything they want, at any time they like. Secondly, some are very active people who may not exercise as such but are extremely physically active. Of course, there is more to it than that...

51

- They do not use food as a comforter when stressed or unhappy;
- They don't spend much of the day thinking about food as they usually have far more interesting things to fill their time;
- They don't usually eat unless they are hungry;
- They do not take notice of peer pressure about size, shape or weight;
- They eat food in a balanced way, to suit their body;
- They eat only until they are full and have the ability to leave food on their plate.

In fact, they view food in a totally different way to us dieters. They view it from an 'Abundant' mindset. They have retained their ability to be in tune with their body and with food. That is, nurture and nature working together in harmony. How refreshing!

And what do we dieters do when confronted by this somewhat rare breed? We express our jealousy; we tell them how unfair it is. We defend our 'corner' by talking about how hard it is to lose weight. We avoid them because they make us feel bad and we never consider what we can learn from them.

Why not stop and look at what we can learn from the simple concepts they use? They have no need to struggle with weight, size and shape because they have an inner sense of their own unique beauty. This is an inner beauty that stems from a belief that they always are and forever will be, 'Good Enough'. They are fully conscious of the fact that love and comfort are not synonymous with food. Instinctively they know what their body needs when it comes to food or comfort and they can distinguish easily between them.

These are some of the skills we have lost. They are the many and varied habits of 'Conscious Eating'. To regain them, all you need to do is start to make new choices and take new actions with food. Practice makes perfect as they say. More than this, it eventually creates new habits in the way you view and use food.

Throughout this chapter you will read about the tools and tips you can use to hone your skills of 'Conscious Eating'. These are offered as choices for change from which to consider the ones that will work best for you. This is how you regain control and power over the food you eat. Through these skills you learn again how to eat to live rather than live to eat.

How switched on are you? Is your head in touch with your body? Following years of dieting many of us have switched off our inner communication system in order to listen to what others tell us. Worse than that we keep ourselves from being in touch with our body's communications. We do this by filling our heads with all those negative 'Not Good Enough' thoughts

So, how often do you 'tune in' to your body and note your energy levels? Your body is made up of energy. When you overload it with too much fuel, you obliterate the effectiveness of your internal energy source. Likewise, when you create an imbalance in the food sources that suit your body, your energy levels are affected. By keeping in touch with your body's food and energy levels, you create the balance it requires. Before long your energy levels are soaring. No diet or healthy eating plan can tell you the exact balance your body needs. Only you alone know.

For a vast majority of her life Sally had no concept of what her body was feeling. The only sense she told me she had, was a desperate need to feel full at all times. As we talked she explained that it was as if a lead plate was placed between her head and torso, deflecting all transmission of feelings and emotions. She had no idea what her body was feeling.

It was as if her head did not have any interest in connecting with her body. To begin with, connecting mind to body was a concept she found most strange. Gradually, by using a short focusing exercise before each meal she quickly began to tune in to how her body was really feeling. To do this she would focus her attention on her breathing, just before she began to eat. Then she practiced being much more aware of the tastes and textures of the food she was eating. Finally, she got into the habit of generating a conscious awareness of how the food made her body feel. Soon she was eating a balance of foods that suited her body. She was eating less and feeling full of energy.

It may feel strange at first to concentrate on the way your body is feeling. Much like an electric dimmer switch, you need to start turning up the dial slowly in order to gain greater light on the subject. Of course practice makes perfect and in this case leads to your mind communicating with your body instinctively. The more you work at it, the sooner you find yourself knowing rather than thinking where your energy lies. This also applies to connecting with how much you are eating.

YOUR FUEL TANK REGULATOR

Most of us regularly overfill our fuel tanks (our stomachs) with far too much food. Either through comfort eating or overeating we put in more food than our body needs. It is then converted and stored as fat. Why do we do this? Because we have an inbuilt mechanism that dates back to our first ancestors and prepares us for feast or famine. This is triggered when we diet.

I would have had no difficulty surviving a famine. The problem, in our part of this planet, is that food is so abundant. We never experience a real famine. Yet, every time you diet and deprive your body of food, you trigger a signal that tells your body there is a famine. This creates a situation where the body works harder to retain the fat. It needs to do this to survive whilst food is scarce. So you are trapped in a cycle of insanity!

By switching on your 'Inner Traffic Lights' (the forgotten signals used to regulate how much and when you eat), you become skilled at eating appropriately. This means not getting overly hungry and making your body think it is in starvation mode or eating when food is not required.

When eating consciously you become skilled at knowing the signals of being full enough. You know when one more mouthful would spoil the enjoyment of what you have eaten. You watch for the signs that tell you when to fill your fuel tank and by how much. For every pound spent overfilling your tank you are adding pounds onto your hips (or elsewhere)! Just think about how much money you can save. I know where that extra money I save is going…

On things that add to my life experience not weight experience!

Before you can use your 'Inner Traffic Lights' you have to be ready to flick the switch that connects your mind with your body. So, it is time to change your focus and leave behind your 'Scarcity' mindset, where you…

- Think constantly about food;
- Focus on other people's needs and not your own self-loving ones;
- Focus on how you look;

- Are self-conscious about what others may be saying about you.

These are the connections that focus on all things external to you. By flicking the switch in the other direction you focus internally on your body, how it feels and how much food it needs. To begin with you may need to sit quietly, close your eyes and concentrate internally on each part of your body. Take your time and do not worry if this feels strange, after all, it is some time since you used this switch.

Now visualise a set of traffic lights, inside you. They are linked to an energy supply created by your hunger levels…

RED LIGHT – Do Not Eat Now
Feeling sick and couldn't eat another mouthful
Feeling stuffed
Feeling very uncomfortable and bloated
Feeling full
Other people request that you eat but you are not hungry

AMBER LIGHT – Think Before You Eat

Feeling physically faint with hunger	These are stages you should not reach as they trigger your body to react to famine.
Feeling so ravenous you want any food now	
Feeling slightly hungry but it is nearly a mealtime	You don't need food yet. Consciously find some other activity to enjoy.
Feeling a little empty	
Feeling neutral	
Feeling physically satisfied	Stop eating
Another mouthful spoils it	
Feeling full but could eat a little more	

GREEN LIGHT – Eat Now
Feeling fairly hungry
Feeling slightly hungry

With practice, the skill of listening to your body will grow. Consciously monitor what causes you to get into the 'Red' and 'Amber' zones. Make notes in your journal or scrap book of the changes you can make. You will eventually notice how much, just one extra mouthful spoils the overall enjoyment of your meal. The best portion sizes of different kinds of food will vary from person to person. So, listen to your body and balance your food in a way that works for you.

Only you will know what and how much to eat by listening to your body. Remember, this is NOT A DIET, so do not get hung up on the quantities. Consider the portion size and remember, your body will tell you what's most appropriate.

Tips To Stop You Running The Lights!

- Eat regular meals;
- Never skip meals;
- Think ahead and prepare your meal to match your hunger;
- Keep a 'Snack Pack' of light and energy giving foods to avoid running into AMBER - the over hungry and ravenous stages;
- When eating a snack make sure you do not eat so much that you are at the overfull AMBER or RED lights by the time your meal is ready;
- Do not nibble when preparing food – by resisting the temptation you will enjoy your meal far more;
- When you are eating keep checking on your 'Inner Traffic Lights' to ensure you do not overeat;
- Eating only when you are at the GREEN Traffic Light your body will not think it has gone into starvation mode. You will not inadvertently overeat. Feel the power of being in control and really enjoying what you eat;
- Eat slowly and with as much consciousness as possible – you will find you notice your fuel tank is full sooner than you thought.

'CONSCIOUS EATING' COPING STRATEGY
There are always going to be times when coping with your inappropriate eating habits will be difficult. It is therefore important to have a strategy for coping - a cycle of thought.

To begin with stop and think after you have eaten something inappropriately. Gradually with practice you will stop and think as you reach for or think about food. The most important thing to remember is that you must never 'kick' yourself for not getting it right. You are a human being and that unfortunately means that you are not perfect!

Think	DELAY when you reach out for food. CONSIDER am I hungry for food or for love.
Emotions	WHY am I reaching for food and what EMOTIONS am I trying to suppress. FEEL the emotion and don't suppress it.
Act	EVALUATE what you want to do about it. DECIDE what choice of action to take. ACTION immediately to heal or fill yourself with love
Remembering	SUPPORT yourself through loving friends and family. RELAXATION is a vital part of the process.
Self-love	REWARD and praise for looking after yourself. LOVE because you are truly worth it.

Remember, **TEARS** are what happen when you eat without thinking! So use this 'memorable word' to help you avoid the tears of inappropriate eating…

The **TEARS** cycle of thought will not work for you every time. However, gradually it will work for you a majority of the time. You can also look for other actions that sabotage your success such as the weighing scales!

Throw Away The Scales!

One of the biggest things to sabotage successful 'Conscious Eating' can be the weighing scale. Let me explain…

I would get up every morning to the routine of the daily "weigh-in". This self-imposed ritual would set the pattern of my thought processes and self esteem for the day. To begin with I would go to the toilet for my first weight advantage. Then I would strip off to gain my second weight advantage. All this so that the weight of my bladder and nightclothes did not affect the final verdict! Next came the vital positioning of the scales. Every room has its 'magical' area where for some obscure reason the scales read an essential pound lighter. Mine was by the wardrobe.

Not content with those advantages, I found a way of fiddling with the settings before standing on the dreaded weighing machine. That enabled me to lose another valuable pound! Balancing unsteadily on the edge of the scales I could reduce the figure by yet another pound and finally acknowledge the weight that greeted me for the day.

As if this warped perspective was not enough, I would then allow the result to influence my day. It influenced the way I saw myself, how much I criticised and kicked myself and what foods I ate. My self-esteem and confidence were dramatically affected by the result of what my dreaded weight machine would say. The negative mindset it left me in obliterated opportunities for me to live life to the full and enjoy every moment of the day.

Talk about avoiding reality! The reality is that a pound or two goes unnoticed by others. By noticing it yourself you keep yourself trapped in a cycle of negative thoughts and feelings. These only fuel your obsession with food. This negative cycle of action and reaction needs to change.

It's Time To Throw Away The Scales!

This can be a scary thing to do. To give up the struggle you must first trust yourself and your body. It knows exactly what size it needs to be. "What if I start putting on weight, how will I know and be able to take control?" Is that your concern? Firstly, the same way as when you lose weight, by the fit of your clothes. This is so much more satisfying and motivating than the ritual weighing in sessions. Secondly, by not worrying about a few pounds! This may, for you, be part of the process of change. If you alter your thoughts, feelings and actions through using 'Conscious Eating' skills, you will create new and more successful habits. These then lead to a healthier, happier and lighter life.

Having little or no idea of how much food was 'enough', Mary felt frightened about giving up the control that dieting gave her. So she used my idea of reducing her plate size. Not only that, she later told me she had bought herself a new and very special, smaller plate and bowl. She explained that using them gave her a loving reminder that she deserved only the best. The crockery formed a visual prompt for her to think carefully and lovingly about what and how much she was eating.

Let go of the old controls gradually and replace them with new positive thoughts, feelings and actions. Remember this is not a quick fix. A slow steady pace will have a longer lasting effect. It also means that periods of weight plateauing are good. Plateauing means the body is settling and stabilising itself ready for the next weight reduction.

If you find you have plateaued for some time and still think you have not found your body's set point, make some changes. Try eating a new combination of foods that suit your body, not eating after 7pm in the evening or increasing or changing your daily physical activity (See chapter 8).

FOOD'S ENERGY LEVELS

Now you need to begin another process of 'Conscious Eating'. This is where you identify the types of food your body does <u>not</u> work best with, as a fuel. You probably know already the negative effects that some foods hold for you...

- The bloated feeling after eating;
- Heartburn and indigestion;
- Tiredness and lethargy;
- Stiff and painful joints and muscles;
- Mood swings and irritability;
- Skin complaints;
- Serious illness e.g. diabetes.
- Makes you feel unhappy.

Some of these may be the foods you crave when in a dieting 'Scarcity' mindset. By making them abundant and allowing occasional, small quantities in your food intake you begin to find the right mixture of fuel to fill you with positive energy. Where the foods cause serious illness find an alternative source (e.g., ordinary chocolate replaced by diabetic chocolate).

Finding the right balance of fuel to create a highly efficient energy source, that suits your body, is the key. Unlike diets that tell you what to eat and when to eat, this is a process of self-discovery. It enables you to determine the types of food that give you the highest levels of energy. Remember, food is neither 'good' nor 'bad'. Food is to be enjoyed whilst providing the right energy levels for your individual body. No one else knows what the right combination of fuel is, only you.

MAKING FOOD YOUR FRIEND

Once you understand that food is your friend you need to take action to make it your friend for life. When thinking or reaching out for foods that have a negative effect on your body...

1 Tell yourself that you can have the food any time you want once you've checked you really do want it, using the 'TEARS' Cycle of Thought;

2 Stop the negative nattering in your head. Remember food is a friend;

3 If you feel scared or in a panic, reassure yourself by thinking how and when you can have the food;

4 Remember how the food makes you feel – reflect on any negative effects;

5 Look for foods that give you high energy levels and make you feel happy;

6 Try foods you thought you hated and see if your taste has changed;

7 Experiment with new recipes and liven up your meal times;

8 Go shopping in exploring mode and find some real 'treats';

9 Feel the energy when you fill your 'fuel tank' with 'high energy' foods;

10 Remember that comfort foods do not give you the lasting pleasure and happiness you are seeking;

11 Treat yourself to the 'high energy' foods you love and let them replace the comfort foods;

12 Remember the physical and emotional pain you feel after eating inappropriately.

SHOPPING TROLLEY SHUFFLE

It takes time to embed new habits and break the old ones of 'good' food / 'bad' food. This is especially true when shopping. So you are now going to discover how to avoid the 'Shopping Trolley Shuffle'. "What's that?" you ask. You know it well – the shuffle as you hesitate at certain shelves that hold your old 'forbidden' foods. It is the internal dialog and battle that goes on within you, as you shop. Or maybe you speed up past certain shelves or aisles in the supermarket to avoid succumbing to the temptation of what is displayed there. Does this sound familiar?

A whole new world opens up to you when you shop in an 'Abundant' mindset. No more shuffling past certain foods as you try not to look. Next time you visit the supermarket look at everything. Take your time and concentrate on how you feel. When you see the old forbidden foods, don't panic or avoid them. Acknowledge how they make you feel. Consider their negative effects on your body and how they do not bring you happiness. Look at them as you pass by. Don't avoid them.

Take a new and renewed interest in what is on the shelves. At the same time keep reminding yourself that you can have any food at any time you want, once you have switched on your inner dialogue ('TEARS' cycle of thought), to determine what foods your body really wants.

As you look at the foods you reach out most for – your comforters – switch on your memories about how these foods make you feel once you've eaten them. Now think about what you can replace them with, as an alternative. What food would be a treat instead of the old comfort food? Go in search of foods that raise your energy levels and make you feel great.

The first time I tried this I found strawberries and mangoes to replace the chocolate I was originally reaching for. That night I ate a great big bowl of fresh fruit and loved every mouthful! I also discovered a passion for pumpkin, a love of radishes and peppers (which I used to hate) and some really scrumptious vegetarian stews.

You are now on a wonderful expedition to find new, fresh foods you have never tried before. Be adventurous by going to different stores, exploring new experiences with food as your friend. Try out your local Farmers' Markets for fresh local produce. Search the supermarket sections you would not normally visit (e.g., vegetarian, organic, gluten free). You will be surprised what you find. You can have an especially interesting time in the fresh fruit and vegetable section.

Make sure you have fun and a great time food shopping. Activate a real love of food as you feel your food fear subsiding. Explore cookery books for new enticing ideas. Keep the convenience foods to a minimum. There is more energy to be found in fresh produce. List in your journal all the new foods and recipes you try and the ones you especially enjoy.

FOOD AND FAMILIES

As with shopping, eating can be a social and family activity. It may therefore have many habits and rituals linked to it. Some of the most difficult situations you may find yourself in, as you change your eating habits, are social and family ones.

Food, especially in families, is used as a means of giving and receiving 'positive strokes'. By that I mean it is used as a means of giving something that is thought to bring the receiver pleasure or make a person happy – a positive stroke. Just consider how easily offended someone can be when they have prepared food for you and you don't want it.

Other difficult situations include social settings, where eating appropriately can make you stand out from the crowd. It may surprise you how uncomfortable others can feel if you refuse a dessert or ask for something different.

Many of these social and family habits can impact in a negative way on the life changes you are making. What you need is a survival strategy to cope with them...

Survival Tactics

1   Know what you are going into – the hidden agendas around food.
2   Think about what you really want to eat.
3   Make sure you are not overly hungry when you arrive.
4   Think about why others may want to sabotage your new behaviour.
5   Be ready to respond to the sabotage:
    - Suggest new family habits with food;
    - Assure them that you are happy and not depriving yourself;
    - Assure them you are not being "good" as all food is "good";
    - Explain that you love them without the need for food;
    - Talk about the changes and why you are making them;
    - Find other ways of gaining 'positive strokes' from them;
    - Suggest other sociable activities instead of eating.
6   Be sure to stick to what you want.

7   Don't feel guilty or play the victim to other people's pressure.
8   Surround yourself with people who are positive about your life changes.
9   Emphasize that you are not being good, just changing the way you view and use food.
10 Feel the power of being yourself and taking care of your own needs.
11 Practice keeping your mind switched on to your body and eat 'consciously'.
12 Consider avoiding alcohol because it can act as a barrier between your mind and body connection.

Living your life using 'Conscious Eating' skills allows you to feel the joy that food brings when it suits your body. It allows you the pleasure of indulging in food that brings you health, happiness and the weight loss or stability you're seeking. The gift it brings is that you no longer allow food to dominate each minute of your day.

The Spirit Of 'Conscious Eating'

Top 10 Tips

1. See food in all its abundance as a source of fuel not fear.

2. Stop using food as a comforter.

3. Take your focus off food and spend your time loving and living life to the full.

4. Build up a sound knowledge of the foods your body thrives on and the ones that give you pain, discomfort or negative energy levels.

5. Keep a focus on your fuel tank regulator.

6. Don't over-eat or under-eat.

7. Use the 'TEARS' cycle of thought whenever you reach out for food.

8. Throw away the weighing scales – both the food and body weight ones.

9. Make friends with food.

10. Use all your senses when you eat and learn what it's really like to love food.

Actions For 'Conscious Eating'

1 Feed Your Soul With...a Weekly 'Dinner Date'

Imagine that you are having a very special friend for dinner –
YOU! Search your memory bank for all the foods you love and
that really suit your body. Find the time to search your recipe
books, then go out and buy the ingredients. Food doesn't need to
be expensive, just enticing.

Set aside the time to prepare and cook this meal and where
possible share it with others. Eat as much as possible in full
consciousness of the look, aroma, taste, texture and flavour of
each mouthful and watch your enjoyment of food soar. Give
yourself the experience of this special dinner date every week.
Where possible involve your friends and family for even more fun
with food.

To find a level of food enjoyment you never before thought
possible, try this 'in the moment' experiment...

- Eat a meal by closing your eyes each time you begin to
  place food in your mouth;
- Do this in private otherwise people think you have
  completely lost the plot!
- Eat slowly and with full consciousness of every mouthful;
- Savour the aroma, taste and textures with each mouthful;
- Consider your enjoyment level when you have finished;
- Eat only until you are just full and not a mouthful more –
  that one more mouthful tips the scales of enjoyment into
  one of discomfort.

The chances are you will have discovered a new level of food
love that you never realised existed!

'Conscious Eating' gives you a new and very different set of
rules to live by. Choose the ones that work for you. Allow them to
form the foundations of your relationship with food. Replace fear
of food with a new focus where love and happiness are at its core
instead of food.

2 Journey Log

Develop a list in your 'Journey Log' of all the new foods that are
great fuel for your body. Create a record of new foods and
recipes you have tried and loved. Use this as a reference point
when you are getting back on track or when you find yourself

bored with the foods you are eating. It is surprising how much you forget certain foods that you have tried in the past and loved.

Chapter 5

The Spirit Of Time
Abundant Mindset Part 4

*Dost thou love life? Then do not squander time
for that is the stuff life is made of.*

Benjamin Franklin

TIME WELL SPENT?

Loving yourself, 'Feeding Your Soul', making the connections and eating consciously all take time. The problem is that old habits and beliefs can hinder your progress towards getting to know yourself and fully connecting with life and food. One of the most commonly held beliefs, is that time is scarce. That there is never enough of it to spend on you. So often, time is taken up...

- Being busy 'doing' for others;
- Working to do a good job for others;
- Thinking and worrying about others and life's problems;
- Helping others;
- Looking after others.

It can appear that there is never any time to focus on your own wants and needs. This may also be linked to a belief that it would be selfish to put yourself before others, even occasionally!

Of all the resources at our disposal, time is one of the most valuable. Like money, love, attention and food, time can be viewed from a standpoint of scarcity or abundance – the choice is yours.

Time is a very precious commodity and should be used most carefully. We actually, all get the same amount of it daily. If we are honest, we all would like more of it. One thing is true it cannot be retrieved or saved by not using it. No amount of money can buy more of it. Once it is gone it can't be retrieved.

MAKING TIME

The 'Scarcity' mindset is like a virus permeating through different areas of our lives. Not satisfied with disrupting our relationship with food and our eating habits, it can so easily gain a foothold in our thinking about many other things including time.

By thinking that time is scarce in your life, you will never feel you have enough of it. If you feel that there is no time to spend on yourself or you are always late, then the 'Scarcity' virus is at work already. Don't despair though. You're about to discover that when you make time abundant there is more of it than you think possible. The key is literally to 'Make Time'.

That's right, you actually can make time. Sounds strange I know.

As a one-time workaholic, I never believed there was any time for me. There were just not enough hours in the day to fit everything in as it was. Trying to give myself some 'Me Time' was impossible. I was definitely wrong on that one!

By making time you begin to expand the abundance process. When you make time for 'Me Time' everything else fits into place with even more abundance.

'ME TIME'

'Me Time' is an essential part of living with an 'Abundant' mindset. Without it you will be sabotaging your success in making changes that lead to your finding the person and weight you were born to be. It is therefore important to know that there are two types of time available to you...

1 **Discretionary Time**
    This is the time over which you have control. When used positively, this time moves you towards achieving your most important work and personal goals. This is where you find 'Me Time', if you take it!

2 **Demand Time**
    This is time, over which other people and not you appear to have control. There are three types of activities in this category...

    ➤ Mandatory - things you HAVE to do.
    ➤ Expected - things other people WANT you to do.
    ➤ Routine - things you JUST do on a regular basis.

A majority of your life can be spent in 'Demand Time' when you don't make time for yourself. It's therefore, no wonder there is no time left for 'Me Time'. This is the special time you take, just for yourself. 'Me Time' is found in your Discretionary Time, which is the one part of time that everything else encroaches on. That is if you do not keep personal boundaries on the time you want for yourself.

So, at present, how much time do you devote to yourself?

"I have no time for me. My work/family always comes first."
"You must be kidding, with all I have to do there's no time left for me."
"Time for myself; that is far too indulgent"
"What on earth would I fill it with?"

I can almost hear these thoughts going round in your head. They certainly went round in mine for a long time. Then I came to the conclusion that no one else was going to give me permission to devote some time for me. Slowly, I began to realise I deserved it.

I started to look at how much 'Me Time' other people gave themselves. I was amazed. If I am honest, I was also quite irritated that people close to me had time to do things I wanted to but felt I had no time for. Then I realised it was not their fault that I wasn't spending time on myself. It was my fault for not standing firm for what I wanted in life - some time for me to use the 'Nurturing Spirit' of self-love.

Not everyone was happy with me when I began to reclaim some 'Me Time' because it affected them. However, they eventually understood that I had a right, just as they did, to focus some loving attention on myself. So I began to reclaim my 'Me Time'. I stole it from the 'Demand Time' and gifted it to myself in order to make those special and important deposits into my 'Bank of Me'.

THE 'BANK OF ME'

Look around and see how much time other people devote to themselves – the gym, golf, sports, hobbies or just some peaceful time alone. They are regularly placing sections of time in their 'Bank of Me'. This is one of the secrets of the P.S. in all we do. That is, 'Perfect Selfishness' - the right to be selfish and put yourself first some of the time. Why? Because there is always an abundance of time if you make it and truly believe you're worthy and deserve it.

By the way, this excludes the time you flop in front of the TV and watch it unselectively. This is just S.O.N.A.R. time (Switched

Off - No Advantage Really). Whilst it may seem restful, it is another way of disconnecting from yourself and life. It is certainly is not nurturing, especially if you nibble on food as you watch.

Each of us has a 'Bank of Me'. This is an account ready to be opened and used. First you have to put into it deposits of time in preparation for spending them. Time is at your disposal and spending it on yourself is such great fun.

Firstly you must plan and set aside the time you need for yourself. Without guilt, you make your deposits into your 'Bank of Me'. By setting aside the time in your diary or on your calendar, you communicate your intentions to others. This makes it a definite commitment to yourself, as important as if you were making time to spend with your very best friend.

Remember, you are definitely 'Good Enough' and deserve to spend some time on yourself. If in doubt, just stop and think for a moment. If you give 100% of yourself and your time to everyone else is that really fair on you? Giving love to yourself is just as important as giving it to others.

You can create a lifetime of excuses as to why you never have time for yourself. You can even allow others like 'Pro' (The Procrastinator) to generate excuses for you – more about 'Pro' later. Constant demands on you and your time can also reinforce your belief that there is no time to spare for yourself.

'Perfect Selfishness' is about knowing that when you put yourself first, it nurtures you in a way that no one else can do. Through placing regular deposits of time in your 'Bank of Me' you will have increasing amounts of spending time. By spending this time on yourself you will raise your self-worth. You will also reduce your stress and find inside yourself a happier, more inner radiantly, beautiful person. What does this lead to? Less comfort eating!

Depositing 'Me Time' in your 'Bank of Me' begins to develop and strengthen your 'Abundant' mindset. It increases the self-love in your life. So, how much time in a week do you feel is the minimum that you can give yourself? What percentage of the week do you deserve to spend on 'Me Time' - 1%, 5%, 10%, 20%?

✓ One hour?
✓ One evening?
✓ Half a day?
✓ One day?

Now let's look at this again in terms of the percentage of time in a <u>week</u> you thought you could spend on 'Me Time'...
- ✓ 1 hour? 0.9% of the week
- ✓ 4 hours – one evening? 3.5% of the week
- ✓ 8 hours – half a day? 7.2% of the week
- ✓ 16 hours – one day? 14.3% of the week

Your journey away from scarcity, and towards abundance, requires you to take time for yourself, every day. Remember 8 hours in a WEEK is only **7.2% of your time!** (Calculated on a 7am to 11pm day)

On your journey to a life of abundance it is essential that you incorporate 'Me Time' in order to really get to know yourself and love yourself. It is in this 'Me Time' that you are able to charge your batteries, enjoy life to the full, find peace in every moment and get to know the person deep within. So if you need to, think again. How much time would your like to spend on 'Me Time', to nurture yourself?

Rachel attended one of my workshops. She had a hectic life juggling a career, house, husband, a four-year-old son and a social life. No wonder she felt that 'Me Time' was a luxury she could not afford. In her mind there was no way she could fit it in. However, the workshop gave her time to reflect about what a great message she would be teaching her son. How he could also learn the importance of doing something special for himself, once in a while.

Seemingly, her small child was so demanding of her attention that this appeared an impossible task but she decided to give it a go anyway. Having spent some time with her son, one day, she explained to him that it was time for her to go and have a quiet candle lit bath whilst he played quietly by himself. Of course at first he was not enamoured with the idea. Then she asked him how he would feel if he was never able to do something he wanted to do? After a short discussion he chose the toys he wanted to play with and let his mother go to have some well-deserved 'Me Time'. That was the start of her reclamation of personal time.

This personal time is your investment in your future happiness and health. It is a simple act of self-love. Don't worry about what you will fill your time with if this is a sticking point. By the end of this book you will have lots of ideas. So how much is time worth to you? Set up your 'Bank of Me' and…

- Begin to believe how much you deserve just 10% to 15% of a week as time for you;
- Begin to love yourself as much as the people in your life that you give your time to;
- Begin to value yourself enough to give yourself 'Me Time';
- Begin to give yourself permission to spend time on 'Perfect Selfishness';
- Begin to put your deposits of time into your 'Bank of Me';
- Begin to think about all the things you would like to put into your 'Me Time'.

Begin to plan time for your journey **NOW!**

Turn to your journal and make an action plan. Every second counts.

PROCRASTINATION

How often do you moan that there is never enough time? Yet if you analysed your day, some of it has been taken up with your own procrastination – putting off doing things by filling time with other actions.

Today is a case in point for me. I have been complaining for weeks that I never have enough time to sit down and write this book. Everything has taken precedence over it. Of course there are many important priorities. The admin work for my coach/mentoring customers has to be done but, if I am honest with myself, I have spent more time than necessary over the past few weeks…

- *Chatting by email with family and friends;*
- *Making coffee and doing odd jobs in the house;*
- *Writing to-do lists;*
- *Updating my diary;*
- *Daydreaming about planning 'Me Time' for the weekend;*
- *Searching the internet for information about a conference that is months away;*
- *Finding housework to do – even though I hate it!*

I could go on, but won't bore you. So, what is it that makes us procrastinate? After all, it's common in all of us. Firstly, it's a safety mechanism that prevents us getting to burn out. Secondly, it's a way of avoiding something we fear or that is strange or uncomfortable. Thirdly, it's a way of preventing change happening.

We do it so that we can prove, yet again, that we are not 'Good Enough' and do not deserve time for ourselves. Considering these facts and that you are very definitely 'Good Enough', all you need is to be aware of when you are procrastinating. Now is the time to make plans to overcome procrastination and steal back time.

STEALING BACK TIME

Stealing back time, how's that for an interesting concept? Stealing back time just for you! Shaving little bits of time from your daily and weekly 'Demand Time', you steal back what is rightfully yours. This includes the times that you procrastinate.

Just think for a minute about where else you can steal time. What about that extra half hour in bed in the morning? How much time do you waste sitting aimlessly in front of the TV? How could you retrieve time from others who get you to do things that they could easily do themselves? What about the times you spend working long after others have gone home?

The more you do for others, the more you raise their expectations of what and how much you can do or are willing to do. Where your demand and discretionary time are out of balance there will be ways of stealing back time. So get creative and start stealing!

DEALING WITH GUILT

If you are still holding back on finding time or 'stealing' it for yourself, it could be because of that negatively destructive emotion – guilt! Generated by fear, it works against your happiness as you allow it to stop you doing the things you want to do. Guilt, never takes into consideration that we deserve some time to ourselves. It only plays on our deep sense of being 'Not Good Enough'. As you begin to focus on the fact that you are 'Good Enough', you are able to make a choice to let go of the guilt. To begin with, lets consider the four types of guilt…

1   The guilt of letting others down.
2   The guilt of being seen to be doing less.

3   The guilt of putting yourself before others
4   The guilt of not doing a perfect job.

Negative emotional feelings such as guilt prevent us from finding the happiness and joy in life we long for and deserve. The choice is yours. Holding onto guilt is a recipe for unhappiness. Allowing negative thoughts, attitudes or behaviours of others to influence you, underlies the patterns of guilt. Spending time loving yourself or planning actions for the special things you want to fill your 'Me Time' with, shows just how special, precious and deserving you are.

I had been a workaholic all my adult life, having learnt the skills from my father. My loneliness as a single parent for a majority of the time (my husband worked abroad and was away for many months at a time) was filled with work as I struggled with an emotional void and the stresses of life. Eventually I decided that this was no way to live.

It was time for me to reclaim my weekends and evenings for myself, yet nothing changed! I continued to work at the same hectic pace for fear that my business and cash flow would suffer. Not only that, I actually had no idea of what to put in place of the excessive work. Friends didn't call me because they got fed up with my always being too busy. I had no hobbies or outside interests. There had been no time for them.

The people in my life were also excessively busy (or so I thought) and so the vicious circle continued. Then, one day I decided and acted on three things. Firstly I made a list of all the friends I could think of. Then I filled the weekend section of my diary with a list of things I would love to do. Finally I picked up the phone and started contacting my friends. Soon I found one who was interested in sharing time with me.

Then I had to contend with the guilt that I wasn't working hard enough. The guilt, that I could not possibly be successful if I worked fewer hours. The guilt of being self-indulgent, of spending time enjoying myself when there was so much work to do. What a load of rubbish that turned out to be! The more fun I had, the smarter I worked and the more relaxed and productive I became within the working day. The more I learnt that it was OK to say no to the work I could not possibly do effectively within the working day, the more I began to live life and enjoy myself, guilt free. As for my work, the miraculous happened. Without the struggle my business grew, even though I was working far fewer hours.

Soon I was regularly planning a weekend a month away with friends or having them to stay. My weekly 'friendship dates' became a joy that opened up new experiences. Friends began to call and invite me to join them. A stream of exciting life experiences and challenges opened up to me. I went land yachting, go carting, to poetry recitals and the ballet. Now I was stealing back time with full abandon and loving every minute of it.

MOTIVATION TIME

Finding time is important as long as you fill it with the positive energy of the 'Nurturing Spirit'. All too often we can fill it with lots of negative thoughts and actions! Within all of us are two 'Talking Heads'– the Negative Natterer and the Positive Persuader. We place these heads in situ ourselves and use them to our detriment or enhancement. How much time we spend wearing each head (because we cannot wear both together) is habit. Luckily for us, we have the choice and power to change the Negative Natterer head for that of the Positive Persuader.

The more we wear the Negative Natterer head, the more time we waste and the more unproductive we become. It will never bring us the joy and comfort we seek. More importantly this is the 'head' that sabotages our positive 'Conscious Eating'. It also leads us into our unhealthy comfort eating. We can wear this head without even realising it, most of the time. Why? Because it is instinctive behaviour born of years of believing we are 'Not Good Enough'. There are, however, a number of antidotes to this powerful and destructive 'Negative Natterer' head…

- Saying YES to 'What is' – the reality of your life. *(More about this in Chapter 7, The Spirit of Healing)*;
- Identifying as soon as possible that you are in Negative Natterer mode and replacing it quickly with the Positive Persuader. *Make a positive statement in your mind to counteract the negative one and start to really believe it*;
- Practicing spending time focusing on the positive, loving and beautiful things around you and in your life. *Count your blessings in life, morning and night as a daily ritual*;
- Practice spending time 'in the moment' without thoughts of the past or of the future. *Concentrate on the beauty and detail of something in your surroundings or take time to meditate (more of this in chapter 7)*;

- Look for the positive in all you do and in all the people you connect with each day. *Get past the negativity and judgements of your mind and focus on the good and positive things.*

As a man thinketh in his heart so is he

James Allen

Replacing negative thoughts with positive ones is a process that takes time and practice. The more you practice the happier you become and the less you reach out for food.

FILLING TIME

Finally, I want to add a word about new ways of filling your time. It can be easier to know what you don't want to fill your time with, rather than what you do want. If this is the case then start with a list of what you don't want. This can prove most interesting! By doing this you will find thoughts of what you do want springing to mind.

Try not to restrict yourself. Make a list of all the things you have always wanted to do in life. Do this even if you have no idea of how you will manage to achieve them or even afford them. Remember, these are things to do NOT to have – activities, not possessions.

A friend of mine told me to write down, at the beginning of a year, six challenges or activities I had never done before. The first year I wrote down 'visit the USA'. I had no money to afford a holiday there, no idea precisely where I wanted to go and no time to go anyway. But it went on my list even though I thought I would not manage to achieve it.

Strange little 'critters' thoughts are! Like seeds planted and forgotten about until spring, thoughts linked to plans and goals come to the surface spontaneously as an opportunity arises. In my case it was a chance meeting with the mother of an American student studying at our local university. Suddenly my written goal turned into a concrete opportunity. The outcome was a visit to Washington and Mount St Helen's before the year was out.

Now I write down my challenges and goals every year. Whilst I don't always achieve them all, I often find new and interesting ones materialise throughout the year.

This process also includes making a 'Happy List'. This is a list of all the loving things you can do for yourself that will bring in the 'Nurturing Spirit' and 'Feed Your Soul'. The list can be as long as you like with things such as…

- Listening to your favourite music;
- Watching a movie/TV programme that makes you laugh;
- Going for a walk;
- Playing with children;
- Gardening;
- Reading an inspiring and uplifting book;
- Spending time with people who 'Feed Your Soul'.

Be creative with your ideas. Make sure they are things you really want to do and don't forget to write them down and keep adding to them. Better still, communicate them to a close and trusted friend. This way you will have made an even greater commitment to doing some of them.

Don't let time or your 'Negative Natterer' head stand in your way. Begin to fill your time with thoughts and actions that bring you joy and happiness. Focus on the joys of each day. Soon you will find your mind revolving to the positive rather than the old habitual direction of the negative.

When 'life happens' and a spanner is thrown in the works, this is the time to use these techniques even more. At times like this the tendency is to spend less 'Me Time'. This is not helpful. So make sure you increase your positive focusing and mental workouts and make the time precious for you.

The Spirit Of Time

Top 10 Tips

1. Commit to giving yourself 'Me Time' regularly every day and believe you deserve it.

2. Create your own 'Bank of Me' where you deposit time for the activities you are committing to.

3. Communicate with your loved ones what you are doing and don't let them encroach on your 'Me Time'.

4. Steal back time and spend it on you.

5. Stop feeling guilty. It is this negative emotion that holds you back from finding the weight you were born to be.

6. Reduce the amount of time you spend with your 'Negative Natterer' head on and replace it with the 'Positive Persuader.

7. Make a 'Happy List' of loving actions to fill your time that 'Feed Your Soul' and then start doing them.

8. Commit to doing six new challenging/stretching things every year that will bring back your zest for life.

9. Take time to be 'in the moment' every day and feel the joy that life surrounds you with.

10. Spend time creating your positive 'Movies of the Day' – positive images of how your day went that replace any negative moments.

Actions For 'Me Time'

1 Feed Your Soul by...discovering 'Me Time'

The fun of finding 'Me Time' is accompanied by discovering new things about yourself. By placing new challenges or actions in your life, you put the fun and excitement into some very special moments.

Make a list of six things you have never done before but would like to do. Make them realistic and achievable and then plan the small steps that will make them happen. If you have no idea how you will be able to make one or two of them happen, write them down anyway. Be open to opportunities that happen unexpectedly. That way, when something happens you are ready to take advantage of a new opportunity. Don't let fear hold you back, just go for it.

2 Journey Log

Make a list of how and where you can make time for yourself. Include on your list the areas you can steal back time from. Now is the time to open a deposit account in your 'Bank of Me'. Once you have written your challenges, goals or happy list, you will have numerous ways of using up your deposits of 'Me Time'. So make sure you continue to make deposits into your 'Bank of Me'.

Only you can make things happen by taking action. Don't just sit there and think about it. Stop yourself filling your mind with reasons why you can't do it – JUST DO IT! Remember small steps are the best. As these are your own goals and plans you can always change them for new ones, as you get more adventurous.

Chapter 6

The Spirit Of Happiness
Abundant Mindset Part 5

*Being happy doesn't mean that everything is perfect.
It means that you've decided to look beyond the
imperfections.*

WHY A HAPPINESS 'FIX' IS NOT ENOUGH
Giving time to spend on yourself forms the first step on a journey
to happiness. Food is no longer your focus or your comforter. The
truth is that sustainable happiness is self-generated, not food
generated. Seeking happiness from external sources, such as
food, offers only short-term pleasure.

Another example of this is where a focus is placed on
material goods to bring happiness. Inevitably, the pleasure of
possession soon dies. As with food, another 'fix' is needed to
sustain the positive feeling. Attaining a certain size, shape or
weight also comes with its down side, if you expect it to bring
permanent happiness. Once the attention and accolades of your
great achievement have passed, it can be hard to retain the
happiness you were seeking in the first place.

Believing that true happiness is dependant on another person
making you totally happy is also an illusion. They can certainly
add to your happiness but not generate it completely. Placing
food, possessions or a person in the position of being the total
source of your happiness contains one major flaw. It overlooks
the receptacle for all this happiness – yourself. Thus you miss out
on a massive resource of happiness generated from within
yourself. That results in a feeling of emptiness. This makes
happiness 'Scarce' in your world when food, people and
possessions are in short supply.

There is no doubt that people, possessions, places and
achieving goals can bring you a 'lift' or 'happiness fix'. None
however, will last forever. A firm foundation on which to place
your happiness is never to be found from external sources. You
can only generate it internally.

This foundation of happiness is essential for sustainable
motivation. It acts as a reservoir of strength when external factors

are in short supply. By creating an abundance of self-generated happiness and topping it up with 'happiness fixes', you no longer need to turn to food as a comforter when external happiness eludes you.

WHERE IS YOUR MIND-SET OF HAPPINESS?

This self-generated happiness comes from many sources. These include all the self-loving actions that 'Feed Your Soul'. It is also dependent on the focus of your mind. How many people do you know who never seem to see the happiness that surrounds them, only the negativity and sadness? This is because they do not realise that happiness is a choice. It is also dependent on what mindset you are in. It might not be your own! What I mean by this, is that there are several mindsets you can choose to focus on...

The 5 Mindsets of Happiness

1. Your present positive mindset – wonderful experiences in the present moment.
2. Your past positive mindset – remembrances of happy memories.
3. Future positive mindset – projection of positive future 'movies' of dreams, goals and plans.
4. An abundance mindset – focusing on an abundance in all areas of life.
5. A positive universal mindset – the wonderful things in the world.

These are the mindsets through which you generate your own happiness. The remaining mindsets are the ones that create the problems for you.

The Mindsets of Unhappiness

- Your present negative mindset – seeing only the negative in life;
- Your past negative mindset – remembering all the bad experiences;
- Your future negative mindset – a focus on fears about things to come;
- A scarcity mindset – seeing things in short supply and craving them;
- A negative universal mindset – the bad things happening in our world;

81

- A perception of other people's negative mindsets – what we presume others are thinking about us;
- A cultural mindset – what society believes and thinks is right or wrong.

When you spend time in any of these mindsets, apart from the first five, the inevitable outcome is unhappiness. Focusing your mind on any of the '5 Mindsets of Happiness' is essential to motivation for sustainable weight loss.

The moment you allow your mind to wander it can get trapped in destructive mindsets that create a scarcity of happiness. Your positive motivation is then lost. From this sad place you instinctively look externally for your 'happiness fix'. For most of us this means turning to food for a 'quick fix'.

It is quite normal to move between these negative and positive mindsets. We can flit between them frequently throughout the day or become focused on one for long periods of time. We rarely stay entirely in one mindset. This is due to the way we have handled life experiences over the years and the habits that we have generated in response.

If we learnt to quickly and easily find positive solutions to the problems that life has dealt us, then focusing on a positive mindset comes more easily. However, many of us learnt to focus on the problem, much more than the solution. We focus too readily on our weight and food problem rather than finding the solutions. This in turn leads to a tendency to revolve to the negative mindsets rather than the positive ones.

Whatever your tendency, the message here is that you can change your mindset – the choice is yours. You can also choose to see a positive for every negative. The key is to stay in the positive mindsets as much as possible, every day. Keeping a watchful eye, on which mindset you are in, is a skill that takes practice. It pays dividends in the generation of a reservoir of happiness.

CREATING INTERNAL HAPPINESS
The more you choose the positive, the more joy and happiness is attracted to you. That's not to say sad and devastating situations won't occur, they will. But how you respond to them will directly affect the degree of your happiness in life.

Some years ago I was at a conference. Two speakers were talking about their different, but equally devastating, experiences of traumatic accidents. Both of them had been left paralysed from the waist down. As I listened to their life-changing stories I was struck by their individual decisions to find a positive way out of their circumstances. Both individuals made the decision to dedicate their lives to sport and not to play victim to their disabilities. They spoke of the difficulties they had to overcome. Yet each one said that, if given their life over, they would not alter the circumstances that had changed their lives forever. Not only had they accepted the 'What Is' – the things they could not change - but had turned it to a positive, using it to form the reservoir of their happiness.

You have the choice to accept the 'What Is' in your life. That is the reality regarding your weight, size and shape issues. Or you can play the victim and fight against 'What Is'. There is no happiness to be found in the latter. So, what are the positive ideas you can focus on to develop your internal happiness reserves?

- A positive belief that you can lose weight permanently;
- Positive beliefs about your ability to make the changes you want in life;
- A belief in who you are deep within, and how wonderfully unique you are;
- Positive thoughts about the parts of your body you love;
- Increasingly loving more parts of your body;
- Positive thoughts about the love you share with friends and family;
- Positive thoughts about the skills you share with others;
- Positive ways of accepting and healing your emotions;
- Positive avenues for creating laughter and fun in your life;
- Using a skill that brings you great happiness and joy;
- Giving of yourself to see the joy and comfort it brings to others;
- Getting in touch with your 'inner child' through creativity and play.

Deep inside each of us is the child we used to be and still are. Time and life pressures may have caused this little child to hide away. On the other hand, you may have just forgotten her or him over the years. The happiness you knew in your early years is still there awaiting the magic of your command to set it free. This is where your fun and creativity reside. The child within you holds the key to another level of self-generated happiness.

Opening this part of you again, may feel strange to begin with. Finding the means to play and be creative can bring old joy and happiness flooding back. Think back to your childhood, to the things you loved to do. What brought you happiness, joy, fun and laughter all those years ago and is no longer part of your life now – games, crafts, toys, art and music? Search hard in your memory banks and discover some of your own, lost keys of happiness.

One thing that children often love to do, that may have lain forgotten within you forty years, is singing. This is such an uplifting thing to do. It never ceases to lift your spirits even if you are tone deaf. And don't let anyone tell you not to sing if it makes you feel full of happiness. Do it alone if necessary but make sure you choose uplifting music or songs. Feel the energy and happiness flood through every part of you as your voice takes flight.

To begin with, searching for 'Little Chrissie' felt very strange and even uncomfortable. Then I took myself off to a large toyshop. This is where my inner child really came to life! Much to my surprise I spent hours choosing one special toy to buy for myself – a set of juggling balls. The thing to recognise here is that you don't need children around you to re-discover your inner child. Your own child is available whenever you want him/her to come out and play.

Some time ago a friend introduced me to a game that she and her sister play, that brings them great fun, joy and happiness. Time together is very special as they live many miles apart. So they often plan time together, which includes a trip to the cheapest store in town. Once there, the fun begins as they scour the shop for the funniest and silliest items they can each find. A budget having been set at the start of the day, they endeavour to spend the smallest amount of money on each purchase.

On arriving home they reveal their items to each other. They play with them, having a great deal of fun with their inexpensive purchases. Tears of fun, joy and laughter are shared all day in their indulgence of their inner children. Letting them out to play is not only fun in the moment but builds a wonderful reserve of inner happiness.

ACTIONS FOR HAPPINESS

It is also in childhood that we establish deeply held beliefs. Some of these are very useful in adulthood (e.g. doing a job well is important). However some are no longer helpful in adulthood (e.g. food is a comforter).

These beliefs are many and varied. They are also personal to each one of us. Knowing they are there and what they are, from a conscious perspective, is important. By being aware of the less helpful ones we can change them for more appropriate ones (e.g., food is a fuel not a comforter).

The first step in changing them is to discover the ones that are no longer useful. To do this you use your emotions and feelings like a sensor to identify which zone your belief is in…

- Happiness Zone – positive beliefs and joyful emotions.
These are useful beliefs.
or
- Battle Zone – negative beliefs and painful emotions.
These are unhelpful beliefs.

When you find yourself in the 'Battle Zone' it is helpful to use some of these 10 'Actions for Happiness' and turn your beliefs to the positive…

10 Actions For Happiness

1. Recognise negative beliefs;
2. Replace the negative belief with a positive one;
3. Replace the negative emotion with a positive one;
4. Find an appropriate outlet for your stronger emotions such as anger;
5. Replace your judgement of others with an understanding of what you can learn about yourself.
6. Remember a positive thought and feeling from the past and reflect on it;
7. Do something that makes you laugh;
8. Stop holding back and start living life to the full;
9. Identify the mindset you are in and make it a positive one;
10. Look for and accept all positive 'Magic Messages', about yourself.

THE HAPPINESS IN 'MAGIC MESSAGES'

Have you ever noticed how some people have an ability to pick up positive messages or loving actions and turn them into happiness? They have a natural ability to feel a glow of happiness when, for example, other people give them a compliment. When someone sends them an unexpected letter, card or gift they are thrilled. If they hear someone talking proudly about their achievements they feel a glow of happiness. When a friend offers loving help and support they feel a glow of love. When others want to spend time with them they feel the deep warmth of friendship.

However, for many of us, these positive actions are just wasted. All too often we throw away these positive messages or loving actions - these 'magic messages'. We throw them away by ignoring them, retorting with a negative thought or comment, feeling uncomfortable or embarrassed when we receive them.

Yet, it is these very messages that are sent to reinforce that we really are loved, loveable and 'good enough'. These are 'magic messages' sent to us as proof of the reality of 'What Is' - that we are uniquely wonderful and worthy of positive messages and loving actions. So let's get real and stop throwing these 'magic messages' away. To do this you need to...

- Look for the 'magic messages' that come your way – there are more than you imagine;
- Notice when you throw away (discount) a 'magic message' and how you discard it;
- Stop yourself throwing them away by giving thanks for them and feeling the glow of happiness as you absorb their magic.

A sure sign that 'magic messages' have been thrown away is a feeling that you are not valued or appreciated. You may also distrust the sender or feel awkwardness or resentment when you give or receive them. Our negative thoughts in response to them (e.g. "She didn't really mean that") also show we have discounted and thrown them away. Frustration or even anger that people don't give you the 'magic messages' you give them is a sure sign you are missing out on many that they do give. This is because to be able to fully receive them, you have first to be able to give them.

Start to give out 'magic messages' to people who readily receive and absorb them. Then watch how they gradually come flooding to you in lots of different ways and from many sources.

USING MAGIC MESSAGES

The secret of 'magic messages' is not just in the receiving but in how to make use of them again and again. It's really very simple. It begins with you inwardly or outwardly offering thanks for the positive message or loving action. Then you retain the happiness contained within them by absorbing the glow.

What you do next though is the real magic! You store the positive messages in the 'magic message' compartment of your mind. This is a vital part of your mind that you need to nurture and develop. It is this part of your mind that has the capacity for instant recall of 'magic messages'. At times of stress or difficulty, this instant recall can be triggered. When life gets tough and your reservoir of self-generated happiness is getting low you can actually replay a stored, 'magic message'.

It is like creating a wonderful movie of the event in your mind. Feeding again from its nurturing power, it replenishes your 'happiness reservoir' right when you need it. Once you experience the power of retaining and re-using 'magic messages' you will want to develop this healing skill even more. Why? Because it is a great way of self-generating happiness.

One day when I was out with two friends they decided to spend the whole day choosing clothes, just for me. They set the rule that I was not allowed to choose any myself. All I had to do was try them on without turning my nose up at any of them. We spent hours and hours of fun as I tried the clothes on and they commented on the resultant look. Their love, enthusiasm and compliments abounded. Never before had anyone spent so much time totally focused on my clothes and me. Until that day I had mostly shopped for my clothes alone, embarrassed by my large size and thinking that only I knew what suited me.

The more the compliments flowed, the more my confidence grew in the new Chrissie that was appearing before my eyes. That 'inner glow' grew and grew. Along with it grew my belief in how beautiful and stunning I looked in all the outfits. Finally when I got to the check out, I burst into tears overwhelmed by the feelings of love that had flowed to me all day. I felt a million dollars and still do every time I wear any of the outfits. And guess what? I never fail to get more compliments from people who see me in the outfits, so the 'inner glow' just keeps on building!

Every time these 'magic messages' are recalled, a glow of peace and happiness spreads through your body. Your sense of personal power, self-worth and self-love are heightened. Acting like a suit of armour, each 'magic message' leaves such an after glow that is can repel negative beliefs and thoughts for hours and even days. Eventually the skill can be so well honed, that immunity to negativity is permanent.

Through this healing process you begin to build a store of positive images and thoughts to tap into. By storing them in your own 'magic message' compartment you have a secret weapon. This positive tool can be used every time you are influenced by negativity – yours or other people's. It forms part of your toolkit for emotional security.

EMOTIONS AND HAPPINESS

The emotions you choose to focus on have a direct effect on your happiness. Powerful, joyous, emotions are your 'Happiness Enhancers'. They come from many areas of your life, enhancing it greatly. Magic messages are just one area they come from, other happiness enhancers include...

Social Interaction

Connecting with people who 'Feed Your Soul' enhances your happiness. These are the people who lift your spirits and are positive and happy. Seeking out these types of people and drawing them into your life is important.

Unfortunately, not everyone in your life will be like this! How then, do you deal with situations where you have to interact with negative or destructive people and their behaviour? Firstly by not expecting them to change – although you can hope! Secondly by standing up for yourself where appropriate and not letting others treat you badly. One of the most disarming ways of doing this is to agree (where appropriate) with the negative comment they have made and throw back a positive and confident statement or question e.g....

"Your quite right, I am overweight! And I love every bit of me!"

"Yes, I am fat and special, caring, talented and strong!"

Create a selection of positive retorts and see how much your confidence and self-esteem rise whenever you use them!

What of the negative people in your life? The ones that revel in moaning and seeing only negativity and problems. You may want to challenge them by stating the positive in response to their negative. If that only makes them more negative (which sometimes happens) then play a positive game within your own head. This is one where you think of a positive to turn round their negative. It is a great game to play without the need to communicate back to them. The effect is that it completely stops their negativity affecting your happiness and joy for life.

Physical Activity

A sense of wellbeing, and for some an adrenalin rush, is experienced after exercising (more on this in chapter 8, The Spirit of Activity). So, your happiness factors can be increased with exercise. Another interesting fact, recently reported in the *Journal of Endocrinology,* is that a brisk walk or exercise straight after a meal stimulates weight loss. This is because sudden physical movement causes a surge of hormones that increase metabolism, reduces appetite and heightens happiness.

High Optimism

The more highly optimistic you are, the less likely you are to see the negatives in life and the less likely you are to be thrown into negative thoughts and emotions. This emotional stability is important. It keeps motivation and appropriate eating habits on track.

Sense of Humour

It has been said for generations that laughter is the best medicine. Now research is proving this to be the case. An ability to laugh every day is important as it aids the balance of chemicals and hormones required for wellbeing and health.

I once went on a holiday where the entire group enjoyed copious amounts of laughter, morning, noon and night. On my return home friends, family and work colleagues kept asking me what had happened to me. I was more relaxed than they had ever seen me, and so full of happiness!

Make it a goal to seek out laughter ever day...

- Connect with people who make you laugh;
- Watch or listen to comedy programmes;
- Read a book that will make you laugh.

And don't forget to share your own fun and laughter with others. Share the happiness within you and see it grow even stronger.

Spiritual Connection

A deeper peace and happiness can be found through a spiritual connection. Through a deeply held belief in a power greater than your own, that has only your best interest at heart, a deep sense of peace and happiness can be generated. Connecting to that deep and peaceful place within you through meditation and prayer also brings a sense of happiness and joy.

Happiness is your birthright so start building more of it into your life now. Discover how much more comforting it is than food!

The Spirit Of Happiness

Top 10 Tips

1. Sustainable happiness comes from a love and enjoyment of life not food.

2. Remember that happiness is your birthright and it is up to you to generate it.

3. Manage your emotions and don't try to bury them with food.

4. Remember that happiness grows with each positive action you take.

5. Make a list of the happiness factors you want in your life and work consistently towards them e.g. to mix with more positive people, to accept compliments.

6. Laugh a lot.

7. Look for 'Life Highs' not 'Sugar Highs'.

8. Use the power of 'Magic Messages' to top up your happiness reservoir.

9. Remember that happiness is found in the present moment. 'The Now', free of past negative issues and future fears.

10. Make happiness your choice and focus in life.

Actions For Happiness

1 Feed Your Soul With...your **'Magic Messages'**
Recognising and using the 'magic messages' that come into your life is a great way of 'Feeding Your Soul'. So it's time to start to consider who are the people in your life that you love and trust. This is very important, as they are the ones who give out the best and most genuine 'magic messages'. Now start to consider the different ways they give these special positive actions and messages to you...

- A compliment about yourself or the things you do;
- Interest and enthusiasm in you and your life;
- A message to say you are special;
- A compliment about how you look or what you are wearing;
- A compliment about your work/creativity/hobbies;
- Help and support in your work and interests;
- All the ways they say they love you.

Remember you are unique, gifted, loveable and youthful. It really is time to love yourself as much as they love you by being watchful for the 'magic messages' every day. Don't worry if you miss some at first, you will catch them next time. Switch off the 'Negative Natterer' in your mind. Don't listen to it telling you that what they say is wrong.

Start to consider that the 'magic messages' may be right! In fact, what have you got to lose by believing them? Isn't it time to feel the positive glow of their action/compliment by saying a genuine and heart felt "thank you"? The fact is you have only your unhappiness to lose and a great deal of self-esteem and self-love to gain. I think that's a pretty good deal, don't you? So start collecting and re-using all the 'magic messages' that come your way and enjoy every one of them as they 'Feed Your Soul'.

2 Journey Log
Write down all the ways you are bringing more happiness into your life every day through utilising any of the 'Happiness Enhancers' that resonate for you...

- Social Interaction – a list of the people who 'Feed Your Soul';

92

- Physical Activity – a list of activities that increase your energy and happiness;
- High Optimism – a list of the positive things you chose to believe about yourself;
- Sense of Humour – the ways you draw fun and laughter into your life;
- Spiritual Connection – the ways you connect with and use the power and strength of a higher entity.

Chapter 7

The Spirit Of Healing
Abundant Mindset Part 6

Any pain that comes is to make you understand the nature of joy more deeply and bring you into joy.

Mother Meera

A HEALING PROCESS

Happiness is a state of wellbeing. It cannot be fully achieved where there are negative emotions and feelings, unless they are healed. Healing is a process not usually associated with weight loss. However, your journey to this point in your life is likely to have been damaging, both mentally and physically.

Your battle with food, a belief that you are 'Not Good Enough' and a mindset of 'Scarcity', will have left their scars. This is a new journey based on self-love, not food love. Here, healing and forgiveness play an essential role in the process of attaining permanent weight loss.

To begin with, you need to acknowledge personal responsibility for past, present and future choices. A different pathway is now required – one with love and healing at its heart.

THE TRUTH THAT HEALS

Beneath all the clutter of our inner thoughts, nestling below the layers of our negative and destructive beliefs, is the very essence of our being. Here lies the truth of who you really are. When you stop for long enough, disregard the thoughts of your ever-chattering mind, you connect with this essence. This is where you find your true inner beauty, love and subsequently the full power of the 'Nurturing Spirit'.

At the core of your very being lies the joy and peace you have been searching for. It is and always has been there, deep within you. Healing and harmony abound when you begin to find the reality that is buried within, reinforcing how wonderful and loveable you truly are. Devoid of false beliefs and messages, love, joy and peace reign. The truth about your beauty and potential shine forth.

The truths and their reality are many, on your pathway of healing. As each truth is identified, acknowledged and absorbed within you, it heals the layers of self-destruction. These are the ones you have spent a lifetime building. It is these layers that have smothered the core of your very being. The love, joy and peace held there are awaiting your healing trigger of release.

The truths are set out here as individual statements. Take time, allowing them to be absorbed within you. Acknowledge the deep 'knowing' of their existence within you. Create new truths for yourself. Disregard the destructive voices that tell you the truths are false. Seek evidence in reality to back up the truths. Look beyond the negative voices and touch the central core of who you are. Touch the love that **Is You**, belongs to you and is there to heal you.

The Truths

- The very essence of who you are is beautiful, made of pure love;
- Your core being is a reservoir of love, available to you always;
- You deserve to be loved;
- Your core of love is abundant, never ending;
- Your body is beautiful and deserves your loving attention;
- There is enough love for you and everyone you could ever wish to share it with;
- Joy and peace do not come from being a certain shape, size, look or weight;
- Joy and peace come from unlocking and sharing your inner core of love, first with yourself and then with others;
- Everyone has this inner core of love. Look beyond actions and behaviour, negativity and false beliefs to find it in yourself and others;
- Through this loving energy you are connected to everyone and everything;
- Food is just a fuel on which to run your body it is not a comforter, LOVE IS!
- Food is not a friend to turn to in times of struggle or boredom.
- Food can never give the lasting comfort that self-love can;
- The 'right' fuel for you is made up of the foods that bring you lasting energy, peace and happiness;

95

- Only you can determine the 'right' fuel by listening to what your body tells you;
- Some foods will work better with your body than others. That does not make them good or bad just the 'right fit' for the purpose of affording you a happy, healthy life;
- Playing the 'victim' to life, food, size, shape, weight or looks is a choice. It is within your power to choose to play the 'winner' and claim your prize of abundant love, joy and happiness;
- Forgiveness opens the pathway to your inner core of love;
- The more you count your 'blessings' and give thanks every day for the beauty, wonder, joy and love in your life, the more you connect with your inner core of love;
- Accepting 'What Is' – those things outside your ability to influence and change - sets you free from the battle with yourself, life and food;
- Life is not a rehearsal so you owe it to yourself to fill it with love, joy and happiness;
- Your body knows when it has had enough food. All you have to do is learn how to listen to it lovingly.

This pathway on your journey is created through the healing acknowledgement of 'What Is'. So isn't it time to look for and accept the truth?

A RELATIONSHIP WITH REALITY

In his research at Cambridge University, Nick Baylis identified that many people distort areas of painful reality in their lives. They find conscious and unconscious ways of detaching themselves from that reality. For some people the process is that of distorting or blurring the reality of loneliness, grief, stress or emotions through quick fixes.

The distortion or avoidance of dealing with the real issue is displaced by the use, in this case, of food. Overeating and comfort eating are the resultant behaviours. If these quick fixes become habitual they can be harmful. What is needed is the development of habits that heal and lead to sustainable improvement in the experience of real life. That is, an ability to confront, accept and deal with reality – the issues that we inappropriately bury with food.

We also distort reality by discounting (not hearing, seeing or acknowledging) the evidence around us that shows we are loved, loveable and beautiful. We discount the reality of what a unique and special person we really are. When your mind is full of negativity and false beliefs, it has the power to see all the things that prove you really aren't 'good enough'…

- You notice the shape and size of others and compare them with yourself;
- You throw away a compliment about how nice you look by believing they only said it because they thought they should;
- You read about others who have lost weight and believe you are a failure.

When you start to heal your life, filling it with self-love, you fill your mind with positive thoughts. Gradually you begin to search for the evidence that these thoughts and new beliefs are true. This is because whatever you focus on becomes your reality. The choice is up to you.

For far too long I tried to make changes in my life based on a negative perception of who I was, what I looked like and what I ate. Many of the things I battled with were futile as they were completely outside my circle of influence…

- *A metabolism different to friends who could eat anything and never gain weight;*
- *A hereditary body shape different to the one I dreamt of;*
- *Many foods I loved that were not the best fuel for my body;*
- *A body shape that had changed with age;*
- *A pear shaped body just like my mother!*

Happiness eluded me as I struggled to change the things I couldn't and failed to see the things I could change such as…

- *My negative, victim attitude to life and food;*
- *Making the most of and loving my voluptuous body;*
- *My habits with food that led to depression and despair;*
- *An abundance of food that I loved and that suited my body;*
- *An abundance of new foods to try and enjoy;*
- *Ways of finding fun and enjoyment in exercise;*
- *Interesting and exciting life experiences;*
- *An ability to truly love myself.*

The truth of the matter is that joy and happiness are founded in reality and in the healing forgiveness of oneself and others. When we are unrealistic about what we can and can't change in our lives we find ourselves trapped. We become victims to a battle that has only one eventual outcome. That outcome is emotional turmoil, which in turn leads to stress and comfort eating.

So it is time to say YES to the reality of 'What Is' and begin the process of acceptance and healing. Finding ways of loving the parts of you that you cannot change is vital to your progress. Changing areas of your life, that are within your power to influence, is the action needed to heal your life and discover long-term weight loss success.

THE HEALING POWER OF FOOD

With healing comes happiness. Have you ever noticed how much easier it is to lose weight or eat the foods that suit you, when you are happy? Along with maintaining your happiness through a positive mental attitude, you can actually stimulate it through the food you eat. Yes, that's right you can really eat to be happy!

It is all down to the foods you eat and their effect on the chemical reactions in your brain. Serotonin is a brain chemical, a type of messenger, that operates between nerve cells. As a natural anti-depressant it can also reduces craving and comfort eating.

So where does this serotonin come from? Well, we make it in our body from an amino acid called tryptophan. Just think of the foods that give you a fast 'quick fix' high. The foods that offer this limited 'quick fix' serotonin effect include sweets, confectionary, crisps, white bread, white rice, alcohol and other processed foods.

These particular amino acid rich foods have a quick release but short-term effect on the body. All, however, perpetuate your cravings when the initial serotonin 'high' dissipates. That makes them foods that increase your cravings as the tryptophan levels suddenly decrease. This is one reason why, when your brain is lacking in serotonin, you reach out for these tryptophan 'quick fix' foods as a comforter. There is no doubt that they do give you the desired boost of serotonin but it is temporary and therefore you are more likely to eat inappropriately.

By eating foods that steadily release tryptophan, the ones that <u>don't</u> give you a quick serotonin fix, you can naturally boost your long-term levels of serotonin. This in turn reduces your food cravings and raises your happiness levels. How great is that!

Maintaining correct levels of tryptophan is critical in balancing your moods and behaviour. It heals the unhappiness or depression that leads you back into inappropriate eating habits. In addition these 'slow release' tryptophan foods give you a long-term sense of well being. If levels in your body are normal, you won't crave or feel the need to overeat sugary and refined carbohydrate foods. Steady, long-term releasing tryptophan is found mainly in…

- ✓ Turkey;
- ✓ Chicken;
- ✓ Fish;
- ✓ Pheasant;
- ✓ Partridge;
- ✓ Cottage cheese;
- ✓ Bananas;
- ✓ Eggs;
- ✓ Nuts;
- ✓ Wheat germ;
- ✓ Avocados;
- ✓ Milk;
- ✓ Cheese;
- ✓ Legumes (peas, beans, pulses, soya);
- ✓ In smaller amounts in potatoes, wholegrain breads, cereals, and brown rice.

Eating a balanced diet that includes some of these foods can help raise your happiness motivators. With other amino acids competing with tryptophan to be absorbed into the body, it is helpful to raise insulin levels moderately to aid its absorption from these foods. This can be achieved by eating small amounts of starchy foods such as brown rice, wholemeal bread, porridge oats and jacket potatoes, alongside protein foods. Sunlight is also essential for the development of serotonin in our bodies.

As a messenger in the brain, serotonin also needs healthy receptors in order for messages to be transmitted effectively. These chemical receptors are built principally from vital fats found mainly in oily fish (such as mackerel, salmon, tuna, herrings and sardine), fish oil supplements, cold-pressed flax and walnut oil.

Depression and negative moods can be significantly improved by daily introductions of these fats, along with slow releasing tryptophan-rich foods, over a three to four month period. How's that for a great solution to healing your cravings and overeating. Eat your way to happiness and the weight you were born to be!

THE HEALING POWER OF FORGIVENESS

Another powerful healing tool is forgiveness. What do we need to heal through forgiveness and why? Well, firstly we need to forgive ourselves for all the times we eat inappropriately. Secondly, forgiveness for all the times we give ourselves a mental beating for not being 'Good Enough' is essential. Thirdly, we need to forgive other people in our life. These are the people who, in the past, have said things about our weight, size or shape that live on in our minds. For some of us they now underpin our lack of self-esteem and self-love. Forgiveness is the channel through which to heal, leaving behind the destructive, negative and false beliefs we hold...

Around the age of 8 or 9 years old, my twin sister and I were taken to London Zoo. During the excursion we had our photographs taken with an orang-utan. The picture had pride of place in our living room. However, when we had visitors my father would point out jokingly that my sister and I were almost as big and ugly as the orang-utan itself! That message stayed with me all my life. It formed the platform for so many of my negative and destructive beliefs about myself.

Needless to say, my father would not remember the incident or realise the devastating effect it had on my self-esteem. The fact of the matter was that he was uncomfortable and embarrassed about having somewhat plump daughters. He never meant to say anything that hurt so deeply.

Trapped in my own mind, the incident's underpinning message grew out of all proportion affecting no one but myself. Forgiving him was a release, for me, from the trap I had created of my own distorted, negative belief systems.

There is nothing and nobody in your past or future that cannot be forgiven, if you are willing. You are also worthy of forgiveness. All you need is to believe that you are 'Good Enough' to deserve it. When others have forgiven and forgotten, isn't it time to cut yourself a little 'slack', acknowledging the need to forgive yourself. After all, your past destructive habits with food were first and foremost a survival mechanism.

This survival tactic now needs to be validated for the splendid job it did in keeping you 'safe'. When other choices of how to survive in a 'Scarcity' environment were unknown to you it came to your rescue. Whilst they were not physically or emotionally healthy options, they were successful in enabling you to cope. They helped you live within the negative environment that life and a dieting 'Scarcity' mindset had created.

The fact is food was used as a coping strategy to deal with all the pain, emptiness and emotional turmoil caused by the bombardment of 'Not Good Enough' beliefs. Validating its effectiveness stops the negative criticisms that lead you ever back into inappropriate eating patterns.

Acknowledging and actioning your growing choices of nurturing behaviours and beliefs form your healing actions. They also allow you to forgive yourself, when, in future times of stress and life crisis you fall back into old familiar habits. And what is the outcome of this healing validation? You quickly and easily move to new and healthier choices that bring happiness, joy and a winning mindset back into your life.

A HEALING RELATIONSHIP WITH FOOD

Healing also comes from facing issues or emotions not burying them with food, or running away (withdrawing) from them. Deep down, you already know how important self-forgiveness is to your happiness.

Healing is about acknowledging your unhealthy relationship with food. When you treat food as a comforter and friend, turning to it in times of trouble, the comfort you receive from this relationship is momentarily felt. Its after effects are destructively long lasting. This is the worst kind of relationship. It does not have your best interest at heart. It creates short-term satisfaction and long-term pain. It stops you focusing and taking action on the real issues that you avoid facing…

- o Boredom
- o Depression
- o Sadness
- o Anxiousness
- o Fearfulness
- o Anger
- o Guilt
- o Helplessness

o Jealousy

o Loneliness

Instead of burying these emotions with food, the key is to take loving action to overcome them (e.g. go out on a 'Friendship Date' to overcome boredom).

If food were a real person would you turn to them in times of trouble? Would the comfort it provides bring you lasting joy and peace? Would you consider their actions loving ones? No! This really is the worst kind of relationship – a destructive one that masquerades as a friend who brings comfort. It is time to end this unhealthy relationship. Say goodbye to it and take action to create new relationships that bring the joy and happiness you deserve.

THE HEALING POWER OF MEDITATION

Letting go and forgiving can be greatly aided by the practice of meditation. If you are one of those people who says "Meditation? I couldn't sit and think of nothing", then please read on. Meditation comes in many different formats and personally I use several of them on a regular basis. Used frequently they are wonderful for...

- Reducing stress and the comfort eating that accompanies it;
- Keeping you calm when under pressure;
- Increasing your happiness levels;
- Solving problems using your inner guide;
- Keeping your mind in tune with your body;
- Keeping a focus on positive thoughts;
- Experiencing the 'Nurturing Spirit' of love and beauty that surrounds us.

All of the methods below aid the healing process. They help to keep your stress at an optimum level (where motivation is high) for energy and happiness.

Clear Mind Meditation

This is a particular favourite of mine for slowing down and healing the 'negative nattering' in my mind. Through regular use of this method you become more skilled in noticing when your thoughts are negative. It aids you in challenging them and replacing them with positive ones. It also aids relaxation and helps to reduce your need to comfort eat.

Find some quiet time when you won't be disturbed. To begin with 5 – 10 minutes will be enough, building up to 20-30 minutes. As you practice you will find yourself spending longer in your meditation. I sometimes treat myself to a full day where I use various meditation methods.

Sit comfortably on the floor, on cushions or in a chair. Sit upright, with your back unsupported – the idea is to stay alert and not drop off to sleep. Though I have to admit there are times when I do nod off! Sitting cross-legged is not necessary unless you find this position really comfortable.

Close your eyes and take 3 or 4 slow, deep breaths, in and out. Focus your mind on your breath, feeling the flow of air passing through your nasal passages. Become conscious of your body and how it feels as you breathe.

Thoughts will float into your mind – this is quite natural - so allow them in. Notice them and let go of them as you focus back on your breath. Feel the peace and tranquillity as you let go. Don't worry if emotions rise to the surface with the thoughts, this is quite normal. When this happens move into the Emotional Healing Meditation, found below.

Clear Mind Meditation is great for using at work or where other issues are 'winding' you up. Escape to the toilet and spend 5 minutes in quiet meditation or better still, find a peaceful place outside. It works wonders! I find it helpful to use my mobile phone alarm to notify me when to end my session. Otherwise I can get lost in time and the wonderful peace that the meditation brings.

Emotional Healing Meditation

This is a really helpful way of dealing with your emotions instead of burying them with food. Using the same method as above, get to the part where you are beginning to concentrate on your breath. Now get in touch with any negative thoughts and emotions. Taking one thought or emotion at a time, switch on your thinking asking yourself "What am I feeling?"...

- Depressed;
- Lonely;
- Guilty;
- Anxious;
- Helpless;
- Jealous;
- Frightened;
- Sad / Tears that cover anger;

103

- Worried;
- Angry.

Experienced in stressful situations, these emotions do nothing towards solving your problem if you get stuck in them. You may even have a tendency to get stuck in familiar negative thoughts and feelings, which then triggers your comfort eating.

The key here is to acknowledge the emotion. The next step is to think back to the situation that triggered it. Trace the emotion and thoughts back in time, where possible. Then ask yourself what you are going to do next to solve the problem that generated the feeling. Quickly reflect on the reason behind the feeling (do not get stuck here) and then construct in your mind a plan of action to either…

- Accept 'What is';
- Find a positive way of viewing the issue differently;
- Find positive, caring and nurturing actions to move on;
- Find reasons why these thoughts and feelings are no longer valid and replace them with new ones that are positive;
- Find a way to forgive the people / person involved.

Then ask in your mind for the forgiveness and healing of the 'Nurturing Spirit'. Once you have experienced the peace that flows through you, when completing this meditation, you will never again want to hold onto those old inappropriate feelings. Finally, take the planned action following the meditation.

If your emotion is linked to a situation about someone else, make a list in your mind of three negative words that describe the person. Use the words that best describe what you really dislike about them e.g. lazy, unhelpful and uncaring. Now, here comes the challenging part. Take each word and put it in the sentence "I am……." (e.g. "I am lazy"). Sit quietly reflecting on each word in turn. Ask yourself about situations when you have been/done whatever the word describes.

Resist the way your mind avoids taking self-responsibility for this learning process. Once you acknowledge this part of who you really are, warts and all, forgive yourself and the other person/people. Feel the release and healing as you end the meditation.

Appropriate feelings are authentic ones. They are appropriate to the situation and form a means of 'in the moment' problem solving. These feelings fall into the categories of glad, sad, angry and scared. Even the glad emotion is useful to consider here as they inform you of what you want, or like, that will make you happy.

However, it is important to identify the negative emotions and deal with them. Holding onto destructive emotions only serves one purpose – making you unhappy. Held emotions such as anger against another person, a situation or where you have an overwhelming sense of injustice only eat away at you, withholding from you the happiness, joy and peace you want and deserve. It certainly has little or no effect on the person or people with whom you have the issue. So why destroy your joy and happiness because of them?

Don't worry if any feelings, around the same issue, come back at another time. It just means there is more healing and forgiveness to be done. Also don't get concerned if there are only tears and you are not sure what the feeling is. With practice you will gradually be able to identify your emotions. If on completing this meditation, the feelings of joy and peace do not flood over you it is possible that there is underlying anger about the issue/person. Where this is the case move onto the releasing anger exercise explained later and then work through this healing meditation again.

Inner Guide Meditation

This is a great meditation when you are troubled with a problem and are not sure of the solution. It reduces the stress caused by indecision and inaction and therefore aids you in changing your patterns of comfort eating.

Follow the directions for the clear mind meditation to the part where you begin to concentrate on the breath. Now visualise yourself on a journey. As you walk along this journey in your mind, begin to see the detail of all the things around you. See the path ahead of you, the scenery around you and in the distance. Looking far ahead of you there is a place that looks inviting enough for a rest. Move towards it and sit down. Look around you again (in your mind) and see the detail of where you are. Absorb the peacefulness of this very special place that you have created in your mind.

Looking further into the distance, make out the shape of a person coming towards you. Watch them as they draw closer. Begin to make out the detail of what they are wearing and of their looks. As you study the kind and loving features of their face, feel

105

the comfort of somehow knowing this person. When they reach the place you are resting (in your mind), invite them to sit down next to you. Sitting together in silence begin to formulate a question in your mind around the issue that is most troubling you. Make it an open question – one that cannot be answered by a simple yes or no. Now ask this true and trusted friend your question.

Once asked, it is time to clear your mind by concentrating on your breath and the beauty of this place you have found in your mind. Do not struggle to find the answer. Wait patiently for a reply to come. This may be in the form of a thought, a picture or a vision of the answer.

Sometimes nothing comes, but do not worry, as the process will still be working within you after the meditation is over. The answer may come to you later in the form of a thought, something you hear or something you read. Watch and listen for it by keeping your mind free from negative clutter as you go about your daily routine. It is this clutter that so easily drowns out the messages being sent to you by your inner guide. Remember that the answers will always be loving, kind and true to your needs. Give thanks for the answer when it comes.

Complete the meditation by thanking your inner guide and telling yourself you can revisit this special place and person in your mind, at any time.

From my experience the answers are sometimes very simple and easily known. Occasionally what comes through from your inner guide is an answer that amazes you with its insight and clarity. One such experience left me incredulous at the solution to my problem. It was so far away from anything I would have ever thought of normally, that I sat there for ages in wonderment at the solution and where it had come from – within myself! The funny thing is, I no longer remember what the problem or solution was. The learning that day was obviously in the power of listening to my inner guide.

Another way to realistically deal with your issues, without burying them with food, is to write down the problem or create a visual impression of it. This way the problem often becomes clearer and therefore the solution is sometimes easier to find. One thing is certain, you will feel a sense of healing just by letting the problem/issue out and taking positive action to overcome it.

Using a healing process is one of the fastest ways of getting back on track with your motivation and appropriate eating. The peace it brings fills you with a quiet and contented happiness. When you have that, there is just no need to inappropriately over fill your 'fuel tank' with food.

The Spirit Of Healing

Top 10 Tips

1. Take responsibility for your past, present and future choices.

2. Focus on the truths that heal. Integrate them within you and fully believe them.

3. Accept that joy and happiness are not found in your looks, shape or size.

4. Create a relationship with reality.

5. Stop discounting all the evidence that points to the fact that you are a wonderful person.

6. Stop comparing yourself to others and beating yourself up.

7. Discover the healing power of Serotonin by eating a good balance of foods that contain slow releasing Tryptophan.

8. Forgive yourself and others and allow the healing process to begin.

9. Use a variety of different types of meditation to reduce stress and negative emotions and enhance happiness.

10. Release any retained anger in a safe way so that you don't try to bury it with food.

Actions For Healing

1 Feed Your Soul With...a process that **Heals Anger**
We can never fully forgive or heal, when anger is present. If like me you were not allowed to express anger as a child, then it can be very hard and scary to let it out. Buried under tears, sadness and even depression, anger can be an emotion that gets 'stuffed' back down with food. Letting it out gradually and safely helps to reduce the desire for comfort eating.
There are a few different ways of doing this...

1. Write a very angry letter but never send it   (or several if needed);
2. Go alone to an isolated place and have a good shout and scream;
3. Kneel by a bed and pound 'seven bells' out of it with your fists;
4. Take a walk and pound the ground with your feet with every step;
5. Take up a physical sport that helps to release the anger;
6. Kneel by a bed, bury your head in a pillow and scream and shout;
7. Imagine the person you are angry with is sitting opposite you. Tell them exactly what you think of them, speaking the words out loud.
8. Find a psychotherapist to help as you work through your anger.

I have written hundreds of angry letters over the years and sat in my car screaming blasphemies to the world! It is remarkably releasing and can also be physically very tiring. The first time I appropriately let go of my anger I was so exhausted that I fell onto the bed I had been pounding and screaming into and slept for hours.

Don't hold onto your anger. It only eats away at you and affects the people closest to you. Its pain and sorrow only causes you to harm yourself further as you bury the anger with more and more food.

2 Journey Log
Make a list of the things you want to heal in your life and the

actions you will take to ensure the healing takes place.

Make a mood calendar in your journal. Mark down for each day, the different moods and emotions you experience, using ☺ smiley, sad or angry faces. Note any patterns and the actions you took that worked best in controlling and eliminating the negative emotions. Note the parallels between the occurrence of negative emotions and comfort eating. Look carefully at the relationship between the two. Use the knowledge that this affords you to continue your healing process.

Chapter 8

The Spirit Of Activity
Abundant Mindset Part 7

The quality of life is determined by its activities.

Aristotle

ACTIVITIES MATTER

Positive energy is a healing force that can also be generated through exercise. Our bodies were born to be active. We need to be as active as possible to burn the food we eat. Trying to lose weight without increased activity or exercise only inhibits our efforts, makes weight loss slower and reduces motivation.

So what holds us back from taking regular healthy exercise? Is it the word itself, exercise? Broken down the word appears to hold the clue as to our issues with it…

    X   For many, this is a negative word that is crossed out of their life;

    err   For others it is full of inconsistency and erring;

    size   For many it holds a size issue.

Therefore, the word exercise can be a barrier in itself. Overcoming the barrier to this word is your first hurdle. By changing the word to 'Activity', already it appears more friendly and welcoming because it indicates limitless choice and pleasure. And that is the key! Every day you have an abundance of choices to increase your activity and pleasure in life. You don't have to go to the gym three times a week to be active and healthy.

What matters most is that you increase your activity, raise your food burning capacity and enjoy yourself. Identifying all the barriers you've erected to exercise and strenuous activity is vital to overcoming them and moving forward.

OVERCOMING THE EMBARRASSMENT FACTOR

Having painful or embarrassing memories can put further barriers in the way of sustainable healthy exercise. These memories may be linked to exercise, sport and games in childhood…

For many years I found I could not go into a gym without feeling an overwhelming sense of panic. No matter how much I tried and persevered, the panic never abated. Eventually I drifted away from each of the four gyms I joined. I felt a failure and yet wondered where my panic came from. At first I thought it was to do with my embarrassment about being larger than nature intended. Then I realised my feelings were not only embarrassment but also pure fear.

Delving back into my memory banks I remembered loving netball, tennis, rounders and badminton as a child, even though I was very overweight. So where did the panic come from? Then I hit on it, an obstacle race at junior school. My somewhat chubby body had been put through its paces on large and small pieces of equipment. The problem came when I got trapped between the rungs of a canteen bench! I struggled determinedly to squeeze through, tears of embarrassment and pain running down my face. The bruises to my chest and back were visible for weeks. The embarrassment and pain of the experience, including my feelings of panic, lasted almost a lifetime!

So what can you do if you are haunted by a negative past experience that holds you back from increasing your body's activity? It's quite simple and great fun. You hold a 'replay movie show' in your head, in a similar way to the ones you use for recalling 'magic messages'. Make it the positive reverse of your negative experience and re-live the event. Whilst doing this, remember to actually feel all the positive emotions that go with your 'replay movie'.

This is a powerful tool to use when any past memory is a negative one. At night, before you go to sleep, try using the 'replay movie' technique. Replay as a positive 'movie' all the things that didn't go so well that day and all the negative things that happened. This is a wonderful way of letting the chemical messengers of positive, happy and loving thoughts flood through your mind and body every day – no matter how bad it has been.

What you definitely do not require, under any circumstances, is guilt, shame, embarrassment and self-criticism. A sense that there is something wrong with you, if you don't like certain types of exercise, is also not acceptable. Why on earth would you do anything (and keep on doing it) if you felt demoralised, uncomfortable or embarrassed? You wouldn't.

Another reason you feel embarrassed can be the effect of the 'Negative Natterer' in your head. I used to find my thoughts really demotivating…

"How stupid do I look doing that."

"I look twice as fat as anyone else here."

"I can't do this as well as the others and so I look stupid."

Or my mind would be full of what it imagined other people would think or say...

"Look at her, she's only been doing this for five minutes and she's already red in the face."

"Why is she here, I know she won't stick at this. Fat people never do."

"Did you see the size of her bum?"

And so it goes on as you fill your mind with such embarrassment enhancing thoughts! Let's get real here. Most people are too full of their own thoughts to be watching what others are doing. Therefore, 99% of the time when you imagine what others may be thinking, the negative thoughts were never reality in the first place.

No one, other than you, caused the embarrassment because the thoughts were generated inside your own head! And if you can put them in, you can certainly take it out again. The key is to turn every negative thought around and replace it with three positive ones. This is a great, fun game that I call 'Spin Doctoring'. You create your own positive 'spin' on the negative way you see or think about your world.

For an even more powerful way of playing the 'Spin Doctor' game, write down your negative thoughts and follow each of them with a list of three positive counter thoughts. It's great fun to read back over them from time to time.

If you are really stuck trying to find the positives, ask a trusted friend for their thoughts. The trick is to believe the new thought. Search your memory banks for past experiences that prove your friend's suggestions or your new thoughts to be right. If there are no past experiences, just believe in the positive thought.

Remember, whether the thoughts are true for you or not, they will still bring you joy and happiness. Why? Because you create your own amazing world through the thoughts you have. Sad, negative thoughts and feelings will always keep you trapped in frustration and unhappiness. Happy, positive thoughts will always reward you with joy. Now isn't that a whole lot better than pain and embarrassment?

THE 'STICKABILITY' FACTOR

If you connect the word exercise with pain, embarrassment or any negative memories, you are highly likely to find it impossible to achieve the 'stickability' factor. This is the factor that is required for consistently maintaining a balanced healthy lifestyle. For many, the word exercise conjures up images of gyms, pain and struggle but it doesn't have to be that way. We are all different, so the first key to consider here is finding activities that suit you.

There is one more factor to all of this, and it is by far the most important. You must have fun doing the activity. If it is not fun, it will definitely not have the 'stickability' factor! This is where the 'Nurturing Spirit' starts working again as you carefully consider the right, fun activity for you.

So, how do you choose the right activities for you? The first way is to consider the types of sport and activity you really enjoyed in your childhood and adolescence. Positive memories such as these make it easier to re-start the activity and help sustain it. When you recall what fun you had, it is all the easier to make the first moves to a new and more active lifestyle.

The second point to consider is developing a creative list of activities that you may not at first have considered as 'exercise', for example…

- Gardening;
- Housework;
- Country dancing;
- Cleaning the car;
- Playing with the children.

That is, any physically strenuous activity you don't normally do on a regular basis. Then of course there are the sports / activities you loved to do as a child. For example…

- Swimming
- Tennis
- Cycling
- Hiking
- Sailing

What about the activities you have always thought about trying but never quite got round to? Considering a life change such as getting a dog is another option. That would aid in getting you out walking every day. On the other hand, you could do your

114

bit for the environment and your health by leaving the car behind and walking more.

Take a nostalgic trip back in time. Play the old music you used to dance to and have a good jig around the house. Even better, do your housework whilst dancing to the music. You won't believe how much fun you can have doing the cleaning! Be adventurous; try something different, or go back to a childhood activity. Most of all get thinking, get active and have fun.

The only thing holding you back is YOU. So get out of your own way and begin to find the 'buzz' and fun in being more active.

FEELING THE ADRENALIN RUSH

For years I tried all sorts of activity, always looking for that wonderful adrenalin rush. That was the 'buzz' I heard so many people talk about but I just could not find. I could get a 'buzz' from my work as a coach, I could even get a 'buzz' from achieving a work related goal. However, the exercise 'buzz' still remained elusive. I even got to the point where I felt there was something wrong with me because I didn't 'get it'.

Then I began to realise that one person's 'buzz' is another person's norm. I had been looking for an adrenalin rush to match those I felt in other areas of my life. For some reason mine was not a 'buzz' more a 'happiness stabiliser'. There was nothing wrong with me. I was just looking for the wrong feeling. Not only does regular physical activity boost my happiness levels but it also reduces the amount of food I consume in a day. Not in a starvation way but in the amount my body actually requires and how much I think about it.

Discovering the activities that create your buzz or 'happiness stabilisers' can be such fun. If you are willing to experiment with new and different activities you can find the 'buzz'. By stretching yourself and trying out different things, exploring new activities, you start to experience new life challenges. New friendships develop, all of which broaden your life, taking the focus away from food.

Hold onto the feelings of happiness, elation, the adrenalin rush or whatever the activity brings you. Don't overdo it though. Exchanging your food obsession with an exercise obsession is just as unhealthy. It can lead to injuries that put your weight loss back months if not years. You may even have to give up your activities for a more sedentary lifestyle again. That just puts you right back in the negative cycle of self-destruction.

So, whenever you experience activity related injuries see them as a signal that there is something for you to learn. If you believe, as I do, that even the slightest injury is an indication of something out of loving balance in your mind or in your world, you have an opportunity to heal it. You can use the inner guide and healing meditations here. Sit with the injury or emotion, feeling it and listening for the small inner voice within you, telling you what is behind the pain or discomfort. Give yourself the opportunity to heal the issue and the injury together.

Steady, regular activity for 30 minutes 3 - 4 times a week, over and above what you normally do is all it takes. As long as it increases your heart rate 60% - 70% above its normal resting rate it is strenuous enough. By keeping your heart rate within this percentile range, your body will be burning fat effectively. A lower percentage increase in your heart rate won't be maximising your fat burning potential. Too high a heart rate increase will cause you to burn muscle rather than fat. So keep a regular check on your heart rate by using a sports heart rate monitor or by taking your pulse regularly.

COMMITMENT FACTORS

With statistics stating that 80% of people, of all shapes and sizes, give up their gym membership within the first 3 months, it just goes to show that we are no different from others. Commitment takes much more than will power. It takes…

- Exercise regularly 3 – 4 times a week;
- An understanding of your motivation enablers;
- An exploring spirit to find activities that bring fun, joy and pleasure;
- Friends to share the experiences with;
- Fun and laughter to make exercise an enjoyable experience;
- Willingness to explore all the possibilities and choices of activities to find the ones that suit you best;
- An understanding of your motivation disablers – guilt, shame, embarrassment and criticism;
- Determination to overcome the obstacles that stand in your way.

One of my friends solved her commitment problem by using the services of a personal trainer. Then she hit another barrier. Her work covers a large area of the country and so she kept missing her training appointments. Rather than give up at the first hurdle, she considered her other options and came up with two that she then implemented...

1. *She and the trainer agreed on an exercise routine that she could achieve when working away.*
2. *She asks a group of her friends to join her and share the cost of the trainer.*

Now there is a group of several women benefiting from the work of one personal trainer. Because of the creative commitment of one woman, in overcoming her barrier to exercise, a group has developed that now shares friendship, fun and increased activity.

Making a personal commitment to a friend who shares your issues, and with whom you can share the activity, is even more motivational. Having someone to meet regularly to share an activity can embed the commitment more strongly. When you are depending on each other to turn up, your commitment level is raised. Furthermore, motivation can be enhanced by a commitment to support each other's positive mental attitude and focus.

Choose a friend carefully though. You don't want one who is so competitive that the green-eyed monster of jealousy rears its ugly head. Over-competitiveness can lead to problems if you appear to be achieving your goals faster than they are. Remember, this is not a race or a competition. It is a journey of discovery, love, fun and happiness. These are the factors that sustain motivation.

Having tried all that, if you still find it hard to stick to a routine regularly then maybe something else is required to enhance your commitment factor. To begin with, try taking the emotion out of the issue by using a multi-focused, logical approach. This may help you focus on loving reasons that can aid commitment. To do this write down the logical health, comfort and choice reasons why you should lose weight e.g....

Health
- Long term and short term health problems;
- Swollen ankles;
- Joint pains;

- Breathlessness.

Comfort
- An end to struggling into clothes that are too small for you.

Choice
- Wider choice of more interesting clothes to wear;
- Wider choice of more fun in your life.

Now write down all the logical reasons why you should <u>not</u> lose weight. Don't bring in emotion – you are only looking at logic here.

I bet you can't find any reasons <u>not</u> to lose weight!

Spirit

But we don't live our lives by logic. The spirit has to be willing. So how do you give the spirit a boost to allow you to follow what your logical instincts are telling you?

- Consider what is the most loving action you can take;
- Take action and watch your 'happiness fixes' increase;
- Consider how you can increase activity, fun and joy in your life;
- Consider how committed you are in other areas of your life;
- 'Turn up' to the activity 3-4 times a week, as if it is your job;
- Take pride in doing your job of increased activity well.

One of the things I learnt when I first began to write, was the importance of 'turning up to the page' every morning. Whether I felt like it or not my job was to write, every day. At that time I had no publisher for my book. All I had was a determination to create a new identity for myself – that of a writer.

Eventually I began to realise that where exercise or increased activity was concerned, I was not consistent. I was not 'turning up, each day' to the activity. It was then that I realised my focus was all wrong. I was trying to lose weight to be a certain size, shape and look. My focus had nothing to do with creating a body full of fitness and energy, in which to live a happy, full and active life.

Whether I feel like it or not I now turn up each day to my activity. My job is to love and look after my body and myself. My determination is to create a new identity for myself – that of an active, energetic, happy woman. Size, shape and weight are no longer the determining factors. They have become the by-product of my happiness.

So, what do you need to boost your commitment levels?

STRESS BUSTING

Reducing stress levels and keeping them under control is a vital factor to your sustainable weight loss motivation. So how much stress are you under and how much do you hold onto? Do you use increased activity exercise to alleviate your 'Over' stress? These are important questions because comfort eating is often stress related. This makes 'Stress Busting' a really important activity.

'Optimum' stress is the level of pressure, experienced in life, which aids you in achieving happiness and success. High levels of motivation and productivity are generated when your life is lived with an 'Optimum' level of stress. This is where you make use of your personal power, utilising the winner within, who stands firmly behind what is right and true for you. An 'Optimum' Stress level is achieved where there…

- Are high levels of effective communication (with self and others);
- Is healthy confrontation (dealing with issues through addressing them or using self-reflection – not burying them with food);
- Is creativity (having fun and time to be creative) and effective problem solving to generate effortless energy, enthusiasm and commitment;
- Is a level of positive pressure of work that stimulates and motivates you into action;
- Is action to move forward towards whatever you are trying to achieve;
- Is a good relationship with yourself, others and with food;
- Is comfort loving replacing comfort eating.

Keeping an 'Optimum' level of stress in your life is achieved through a consistent balance of positive thoughts and emotions and regular physical activity. The more happiness and joy you generate through activity, personal responsibility and self-awareness, the more consistent your 'Optimum' level of stress will be.

The problem is, the levels of pressure people need to attain 'Optimum' Stress varies from person to person. Accompanying this is the problem that the difference between 'Optimum Stress' and 'Over Stress' is a very slim one. The impact of your work and life-style can therefore tip the balance towards 'Over' Stress without you realising it.

Consequently, you need to be aware of the signals that identify when you have tipped the scales from 'Optimum' Stress to 'Over' Stress. These signals differ from person to person. They may include things such as poor or reduced communication levels, a reduced ability to solve problems, unhappiness, depression, illness, irritability, insomnia, panic attacks, tension, headaches, forgetfulness or withdrawal from being with people.

'Over' stress is often brought on by a combination of work and personal pressures. Action is therefore required to keep a balance of 'Optimum' Stress. Other people can easily contribute to your 'Over' stress levels. Like us, others can be well into 'Over' Stress without even realising it. These people are the stress carriers!

As with any illness, the trick is to catch it before it takes hold and spreads from one person to another, especially before it spreads to you. The first step is to identify if you are a stress carrier and then take action to return to a state of 'Optimum' Stress...

- Consider and list the issues, people or circumstances that are influencing your over stress;
- Taking each issue at a time, consider if it is within your circle of influence to take action;
- Where the answer is no or not at the moment it is up to you to let go of the issue, as it is affecting you negatively and causing you to be a stress carrier;
- If the answer is yes, consider what action you can take to overcome the problem / issue and take action on it.

The very fact that an action is taken aids in the reduction of stress. It is inaction and holding onto the things you have no power to influence that cause your stress levels to increase. Letting go and accepting the things you cannot influence is vital to the process of reducing your stress and comfort eating.

The more you are content in the roles you play and the work you do, the more you will align with your 'Optimum' stress levels. Some of your stress levels come from people and external factors. Often these can be the unexpected, negative situations that you may or may not have an influence over.

Consider for one moment the negative impact that other people who are stress carriers have on you. Wouldn't it be nice to build a cocoon around you so that the bombardment of their stressful, negative energy does not affect you? Well you can!

Just as happiness is a choice, so is achieving 'Optimum' Stress. Think of stress as ball of fire that evokes negative emotions. When you are with stressed people they throw their balls of fire out into the ether for anyone to catch. They do this by moaning or using negative, aggressive emotions and words. Catching these balls of fire – 'Stress Balls' - is often instinctive or habitual. You can, if you choose, decide not to catch them. To be able to do this there are 5 key questions to ask…

1. Is this person's behaviour coming from a level of over stress?
2. Does this stress belong to me in any way, shape or form?
3. Am I absolutely certain the reason for their stress belongs to me?
4. How can I understand their fears and empathise with their stress?
5. What can I say or do that allows me not to pick up their 'Stress Ball' and have them affect me?

Consider a recent stressful situation that you were in which involved interaction with another person. The reality is that their stress did not belong to you. It is owned by them and is highly likely to be generated from their own personal fears. Now…

✓ Ask yourself the first three questions above.
✓ Carefully consider what their fear might be and answer question 4
✓ A simple statement such as "I can see how difficult this is" can easily stop you from catching the 'Stress Ball' yourself whilst helping to reduce its effect on the other person.
✓ If their stressful reaction is unacceptable you can always close down the communication by saying that you will be willing to talk things through when they have calmed down.
✓ On the other hand, if their stressful reaction has caused them to put you down or be offensive, you can make a strong statement such as "That is not acceptable! I will not be spoken to like that."

This enables you to hold onto your personal power whilst at the same time not picking up the other person's 'Stress Ball'.

When you do catch these balls of destruction, they can affect so much more of your day, not just the moment it happens...

Most nights on her way home from work, one of my clients would get more and more wound up about the rush hour traffic and the state of other people's driving. By the time she reached her home and family she was usually so wound up that the evening would be full of negativity, arguments and of course comfort eating. All she wanted was some space and time to chill out and be alone to unwind from work. Instead she got home to be confronted by more work and hassle!

Her children and husband could be forgiven for thinking that they were the cause of her stress and negativity. In fact her stress was generated from a combination of work frustrations and other people's stress. She ended each day holding onto numerous 'Stress Balls'. Then she would fling them at everyone when she got home. Inevitably, most of the time others caught them and a battle of the 'Stress Balls' resulted.

She began to examine the accumulation of multiple 'Stress Balls', picked up during her working day. Then she realised how she became the 'Stress Carrier' to her family.

Her decision to let go of her stress, before arriving home, had an interesting angle to it. Looking forward to, and enjoying, the traffic delays was her solution! This was one of her stress accumulators and she turned it into her stress reliever. Why? Because it gave her more time to listen to her favourite music, notice the beauty around her and let go of the events of the day. The result was no more 'Stress Ball' fights with the family. The benefit, an increased happiness factor from quality time with the ones she loved.

Working at reducing the number and effect of the 'Stress Balls' in your life is another great way of reducing your level of comfort eating. At the same time it will increase your happiness factors.

STRESS TRIGGERS

Knowing and understanding your 'Stress Triggers' is also a vital part of the process of stress reduction. The triggers are many and varied but usually you will find a pattern to them, in your life. The same people/types of people or situations can crop up time and time again in our life. Until you learn to view them and handle them differently they have an uncanny knack of reappearing. Altering how you respond to stress triggers breaks their hold over you and sets you free. Some of the areas to consider which may hold 'Stress Triggers' for you are…

- People you resent;
- Jealousy;
- Held anger;
- Personality clashes;
- Work areas you are under confident about;
- High pressure work that does not match your 'Optimum' stress pressure levels;
- Work that does not give you job satisfaction;
- Injustices done to you or others;
- Other people who manage or treat you in a negative way;
- Situations that produce high levels of fear;
- Change or unpredictability.

Creating new ways of viewing different situations is a process of reframing. This allows you to alter your response and therefore reduce your stress levels. Reframing the situation in your mind so you can take positive action is the objective. Letting go of the negative and focusing only on the positive, can be a hugely effective stress reliever.

There are three steps in this process of reframing the issue…

1 Decision
2 Action
3 Letting go

1 Decision

Before making a decision about the situation, consider the following…

✓ What or who is influencing the situation?
✓ Whose head is your thinking inside – are these your thoughts or another person's thoughts or assumptions of other people's thoughts?
✓ What resentments and anger are you holding onto?

Your mind wants to prove you right and the other person wrong. This is where a lot of stress lies. In reality, considering that each person views their world from different perspectives, both opinions may well be right. In fact other people's attitudes and the situations you find yourself in are really your learning opportunities.

"What is she on about?" I can hear you ask. Consider for a moment that every person in the world is responsible for his or her own thoughts, feelings and actions. These are what make up their perception of the world they live in. Battling with others to get them to change their view of the world, to match your own, can be not only futile but also destructive and highly stressful!

The battle to change other people's view of the world, inevitably causes some of the 'Stress Triggers' in your life. Accepting that the other person's reality may not match yours and they may never see things your way, creates new and less stressful choices for you to consider. These situations can teach you more about tolerance and unconditional love.

2 Action

The actions you take in these 'Stress Trigger' situations can either increase your stress or increase your happiness. The choice is yours but it does not entail being submissive and backing down – that only builds resentments. Your choices of action are therefore to...

- ✓ Accept that there is nothing you can do to change the person or situation;
- ✓ Acknowledge the other person's right to see the world from their perspective and walk away having agreed to differ;
- ✓ Acknowledge that what they say about you may well be right from their perspective;
- ✓ Consider what you can learn about yourself by accepting the situation;
- ✓ Consider how you can be grateful to the person or for the situation;
- ✓ Give thanks mentally for this learning experience;
- ✓ Consider how you have reduced your stress and levels of comfort eating and praise yourself for such an achievement.

3 Letting Go

The final stage is to let go of your need to be right or justified. By doing this you let go of the battle and the stress. This can be done by...

- ✓ Accepting the situation and working with it using an open and loving heart;
- ✓ Accepting that which is outside your circle of influence to change;
- ✓ Accepting that everyone has the right to see things from their own perspective;

✓ Accepting responsibility for doing what is kind and loving, given the situation;

✓ Accepting that difficult people and situations provide wonderful learning opportunities.

You reduce your stress levels when you learn to accept and love 'What Is'.

Stress Relieving

There is only one thing that relieves stress and that is action. These are the actions of acceptance and letting go. The actions of 'Feeding Your Soul' and increasing physical activity. These all raise positive energy and reduce stress. The actions of 'Feeding Your Soul' with self-love raises happiness and reduces stress. The action of replacing negative thoughts and feelings with positive ones increases happiness and reduces stress. The action of forgiveness and healing lets go of resentments and reduces stress. The action of accepting 'What is' stops your battle with the things you can't change and reduces stress.

All these actions have just one outcome – comfort eating and inappropriate food intake are dramatically reduced. This happens without any shame, guilt or self-loathing. How wonderful is that! So activate your power for action activity exercise as many times as possible every day. Discover where your potential for happiness and 'Optimum' Stress really lies. Make increased activity fun and an integral part of your life.

The Spirit Of Activity

Top 10 Tips

1. Use the 'Green Gym' – the natural world – as much as possible. It's free!

2. Work with people who enjoy having fun while taking regular exercise.

3. Remember, it takes fun to create the 'Stickability' factor.

4. Start to love your job of taking increased activity.

5. Don't do your physical activity alone unless you really want to. It can be far more fun and supportive to be active with others.

6. Be adventurous, try out new activities, join some different groups or classes.

7. Share the cost of a personal trainer if it helps you stick to a regular routine.

8. Search for your 'Adrenaline Rush' or 'Happiness Stabiliser' and focus on how good it makes you feel.

9. Measure all the different parts of your body and re-measure every month (No more often). This can be far more motivational than jumping on the scales every day!

10. Be prepared for the boredom factor to kick in at some stage. Have a few more activities ready to try out when you need a change. Don't just give up all activity.

Actions For Activity

1 Feed Your Soul With...your **Activities for Fun**!

Start to explore the activities that most attract you. Don't forget the importance of using the 'Green Gym' – the beautiful, natural world around you – it is free! Have fun finding and using the activities that make you feel great. Share your experiences with friends. Start an activity group. Someone in the group may open your eyes to new and exciting activities.

Don't discount the gym or other activities you have tried in the past. Explore as many activities as you want until you find the few you feel inspired to commit to. Always have a reserve list. This is for the times when injury or boredom creep in and the 'Stickability' factor begins to wane. Then you will always have new and fun activities to switch to quickly and easily.

2 Journey Log

In your journey log make a list of all the criteria that you know will help you commit, long term, to regular activity that will increase your heart rate by 70%. If you find that difficult, begin with a list of what you definitely don't want and then move to writing about what you do want.

Make a list of all the sport and exercise you have done in the past. Rate them each on a scale of 1 – 10 for their enjoyment factor (where 10 is the top score). Now prioritise which ones you want to have a go at again, making sure they match your criteria. Also make a list of activities you have never tried and score/rate them for their interest level in the same way. Combine the two lists. Now you have your activity plan. Go for it!

Chapter 9

Finding Your Full Potential

As a being of Power, Intelligence and Love, and the Lord of his own thoughts, man holds the key to every situation, and contains within himself that transforming and regenerative agency by which he may make himself what he wills.

James Allen

FULFILLING YOUR POTENTIAL

Somewhere deep inside is the person you really are, waiting to get out. You know the one. They have great potential, beauty, attractiveness and confidence in how they look. They love the person they are, the body they live in and the life they lead

Finding that person is the journey I took. Now as you finish reading this book, I hope you will too. What a journey it can prove to be, interesting, exciting, challenging and full of new experiences and people. There is never a dull moment. And the remarkable thing is, its focus is not on food but on the 'Nurturing Spirit' of self-love. Yet, you can still lose weight!

Each of us has the potential, deep within, to be far more than we ever imagined possible. We can go further, achieve more and find the weight we were born to be. What prevents you from achieving these desires is fear and its subsequent negative messages. So the challenge is to begin your journey to a new 'Abundant' mindset by developing your potential to...

- Let go of shame, guilt, fear and self-loathing;
- Live each day in happiness and joy;
- Change your negative thoughts and beliefs for positive ones;
- Love yourself more than anyone else can ever do;
- Focus on your 'blessings', giving thanks for them constantly;
- Accept 'What Is' by turning it into 'What I need to learn';
- Love your body image as it is each day;
- Link vision and emotion to create your dreams;
- Use your 'conscious eating' skills every day;
- Fuel your body to find its highest energy levels;

- Activate yourself, keeping stress at bay, stopping comfort eating.

As I said at the start of this book, changing your mindset is a matter of choice. Success comes from commitment to daily practice. It is not hard. All it takes is tenacity to keep challenging the negative to change beliefs and behaviours. By focusing on 'Conscious Eating', increased activity and the vision of yourself as a happy, joyful person you will find the weight you were born to be.

Now that you have almost finished reading this book, the time has come to overturn your negative images, issues and fears. It is time to take some life-changing actions or consolidate the ones you have already started.

BODY IMAGE

Life-changing accomplishments may be short-lived if the actions to achieve them are not matched by the way you think. Your body shape may change, with increased activity and eating food that suits your body. But how do you shape your body image? By that I mean, the way you love and think about your body. How do the positive effects of your conscious eating and regular healthy activity match the way you think about your body?

This is a dilemma for many, and one you may still be struggling with. Loving every part of your body, even the 'wobbly bits', can be a challenge. Yet, it is essential to your sustained motivation and permanent weight loss. Success is linked to your ability to achieve a positive body image, no matter what size, shape or weight you are.

The fear is, that if we have a positive body image when we are overweight we would not be motivated enough to lose weight. What rubbish! You lose weight because you love your body and want to be happier and healthier, not because you hate it.

When you exercise and diet because you hate your body the chances are, when you lose weight, you will still not love your body image. This frustration and dissatisfaction with your body is one of the major reasons why, when you reach your target weight, you are still not happy. Inevitably the motivation goes and the weight creeps back on.

Not loving every part of your body can lead to you having a distorted perception of it. Many of us have a perceived body image that we think is far bigger than it really is. If asked to assess our size against others, many of us see ourselves as three or four times bigger than we actually are.

When I began to lose weight from my massive size 30, it took months for my friends and family to persuade me that I needed to buy new clothes. Even when my daughter kept telling me that my clothes were hanging off me, it did not register. When I looked in the mirror – which wasn't often in those days – all I saw was a fat woman. I never acknowledged that my clothes were loose and baggy on me!

Eventually common sense prevailed and I went shopping. What amazed me was that an outfit a size smaller (28) was too big, a size 26 was still too big and a size 24 fitted perfectly. I had been wearing clothes 3 sizes too big for me! I had been pinning them up at the waist and still my mind did not register the reality of my new body image. Only when I saw myself in the new clothes did the veil of self-deception fall from my eyes.

So why do we find it difficult to love our bodies and see them as they really are? Is it because when we are so fixated on a world of size, weight and shape issues, that shame and guilt smother our ability to love ourselves? Do these negative emotions create such a strong self-hatred that we are unable to find it in our hearts to love ourselves as we really are?

Without accepting the reality of your true body shape and size you are trapped, forever believing you are 'not good enough'. Even when you achieve the weight you were born to be, this dissatisfaction could still prevail. Without a true loving and positive body image you will never be happy, no matter what weight you are!

Without a love of your body you will be increasing your levels of stress every time you see your body, or think about it with shame and loathing. When you truly love someone, you learn to love every part of them and accept their foibles and idiosyncrasies. It really is time to start believing that you deserve this level of unconditional love, from yourself, right now!

Your body is the vessel you were given to live your life within. Love it for what it is. Love it for the lessons it offers in how to give unconditional love. Love it for the lessons it offers in how to live life to the full, embracing all the love that surrounds you. Finally, love it because all it wants is to sustain you in a happy, healthy and joyful life. Let it do its job; listen to what it needs from you – the 'Nurturing Spirit' of love and activity – and learn to truly love it.

ROLE MODELS

Some time ago I was with my father watching guests arrive at a hotel for a wedding. A comment made by my father drew my attention to a very large lady. "Good God, just look at the size of her!" he exclaimed. As I looked at her my mind was full of thoughts like "She is huge and looks just awful in that dress." "Why doesn't she realise how big she is and do something about it?" "Just look at the size of her bottom."

Then I remembered a quote I read some time ago...

If you want to know what you think of yourself, ask yourself what you think of others and you will find the answer.

Seth

In that moment I looked at the woman again, studying her with love and not judgement. New thoughts began to generate from my altered mindset – "She looks stunning in that colour outfit." "Her happiness and love radiate for all to see and people are drawn to her warmth." "How lovely and cuddly she is." That was the moment I really began the final process of loving myself. Now, the more I replace my negative judgement of large people with caring, loving thoughts, the more I learn to totally love my own body image.

By viewing other large men and women with loving kindness and positive thoughts, we begin to build a positive body image of ourselves. We begin a process of self-acceptance as we more readily accept others. This in turn increases our self-love, as we choose happiness and the fuels that feed it.

Not only does it take tenacity to keep motivation levels high but it also takes an ability to truly love yourself and your body. Having role models to identify with is therefore important. I am not talking about thin trim super models or celebrities here. I am talking about large voluptuous men and women. These are the ones who are confident, sexy, spirited, active and living life to their full potential. Dawn French springs to mind for me. If you have ever watched her in a live performance, racing around the stage, you will know what I mean. When we identify with large men or women and acknowledge the parts of their characters

131

and body that we love, we are actually giving permission to accept and love ourselves in that way.

When I admire Fern Britton for her skills as a presenter and her joy of life, I am connecting to that part of me that loves myself enough to know I have the same potential. When I watch Dawn French in a physically active role, I feel inspired by her energy. When I watch her being photographed draped in muslin like a Ruben's model, sexy and voluptuous, it reinforces for me that no matter what my size, I am attractive and desirable.

It is the well-known demons of fear, guilt and shame that hold us back from loving ourselves and our bodies as they are right now. There is no one in the world who doesn't face his or her own inner demons and fears at some stage. However, some people are just more programmed than others to focus on their fears and negativity. That doesn't mean that those fears and negativity are insurmountable. Confronting and overcoming them demonstrates the power of personal potential, once fear is faced and triumphed over.

One remarkable young man, at the age of just 21, was diagnosed with Motor Neurone Disease. This is a degenerative disease of the nerve cells of the body. He was told that it would affect every part of his body except his brain. It would render him unable to move, talk and eventually breathe. Finally it would lead to an early death within, at best, a couple of years. The man was Steven Hawking, whose brilliant mind has changed the world's perception of time and space. Today, over 40 years on from the diagnosis of a terminal illness, he is still working even though he is unable to move or talk in the conventional way.

How many people can you think of whom you admire for their tenacity, courage and fearlessness? How many people do you know who inspire you by the way they lead their lives or have overcome adversity? Make a list of all the characteristics you admire about them. This is a useful way of finding the same resources within yourself. These people are actually no different from you. All that is different is that you may not have tapped into these inner resources as yet.

How many large and wonderful people can you think of as role models? Start to build your list and look on them with love and not judgement.

YOUR BELIEFS CREATE YOUR POTENTIAL

It is not just how you see yourself that can hold you back. What you believe about yourself and your world can either propel you forward towards your potential or hold you back in life. If you believe 'I can't'; I shouldn't'; 'I don't have the skills, talent or ability' etc., these messages will form the root of your self-limiting beliefs. They are all blocks to your potential. Your negative beliefs create your reality until you choose to let them go and start moving towards your potential by believing the truth...

You are unique, perfect, wonderful, powerful, gifted, whole, strong, loving, harmonious and happy

If you believe that your weight and size hold you back from living life to the full, then that is the reality you will create. Finding the weight and size you were born to be becomes possible, when you start loving yourself enough to believe in your ability to change your life.

These words of Nelson Mandela say it all...

Our deepest fear is not that we are inadequate.
Our deepest fear is that we are powerful beyond measure.
It is our light not our darkness that frightens us.
We ask ourselves,
"Who am I to be; brilliant, gorgeous, talented and fabulous?"
Actually, who are you not to be?
You are a child of God.
Your playing small doesn't help the world.
There is nothing enlightened about shrinking so that others will not feel insecure around you.
We were born to manifest the glory of God that is within us.
It is in everyone.
It is not just in some of us.
And as we let our own light shine we unconsciously give permission to others to do the same.
As we are liberated from our own fear our presence automatically liberates others.

Nelson Mandela - from his 1994 inaugural address

The more you project positive images of yourself, linked to joyful, loving and excited emotions, the more you dissipate your negative ones. You allow your potential to blossom. Follow your instinct, your inner guide. Let it guide you in how you live your life, what you eat and how you find your potential.

THE POWER OF BOUNDARY SETTING

Achieving your potential and your weight loss goal requires a game plan – a set of boundaries. All game plans require a strong set of rules for success. This process is no different. Boundaries (rules, standards, realistic expectations and achievable goals) form the foundation of your game plan. They are very different from the dieting game plan and therefore require you to build new rules and boundaries.

Boundaries need to be well set. When clearly stated they allow for good positive feedback when they are being met. They also act to aid learning when the boundaries begin to slip. Unlike dieting, where criticism, peer pressure, guilt and shame are the tools that reinforce the boundaries of a 'Scarcity' mindset, an 'Abundant' mindset is built on a framework of loving actions. These self-chosen boundaries underpin the success of your goals. They provide a foundation on which to base self-questioning and self-reflection techniques.

The boundaries of an 'Abundant' mindset are therefore used as an effective learning and motivation tool. That makes them much more useful than the self-criticism of a 'Scarcity' mindset. This self-reflective approach facilitates learning. It allows for the positive reframing of beliefs and behaviours rather than the familiar rebellion caused by criticism and a belief that you have failed.

You know, all too well, the damaging effect of being told by yourself or others that you are 'not good enough'. This happens when the rules of your diet or exercise routine are broken. Self-reflection, on the other hand, reinforces the fact that you are doing well in many other ways. It can remind you that it is only human nature to err and that a boundary or rule broken is an opportunity to learn and move forward.

So how does self-reflection work? Firstly you need to develop your own list of boundaries and rules about the food you eat, the thoughts and beliefs you focus on and the physical activity you take. Forget the old boundaries of your 'Scarcity' mindset. It is time for you to set new rules that are applicable only to you.

When I settled down to write my own set of boundaries, I realised that by putting them down on paper they increased my commitment to taking responsibility for myself. No longer did I have a list of rules, with which I could beat myself up. These were rules by which to live, learn and praise myself. I chose them because they enabled me to...

> - *Eat a predominance of foods that give me a high level of energy (because it makes me happier);*
> - *Eat a minimal amount of red meat and fatty foods (because they give me indigestion);*
> - *Eat more vegetarian food with some fish and chicken (because they give me more energy and no joint pains);*
> - *Eat fresh rather than processed foods (because they give me energy and reduce that bloated feeling);*
> - *Eat minimal amounts of carbohydrates and sweet foods (because they give a Serotonin 'high' and trigger my food craving);*
> - *Eat only when I am hungry and then only until I am just full (because I gain a higher level of food enjoyment);*
> - *Replace comfort eating with comfort loving - actions that 'Feed My Soul' (because it makes me feel so happy and loved);*
> - *Do my meditation every day (because it reduces my comfort eating and brings me peace and joy);*
> - *Take 30 minutes of physical activity that raises my heart rate. Do this at least 3 times a week (because it increases my energy and happiness levels);*
> - *Notice negative thoughts and replace them with positive ones (because it helps me see the reality I normally discount);*
> - *Keep track of which mindset I am in and keep refocusing on the positive ones (because they build my reservoir of happiness);*
> - *Count my blessings first thing in the morning and last thing at night (because it begins and ends each day with a feeling of joy);*
> - *Use my creativity every day, especially through my writing (because it never fails to lift my spirits & keeps my motivation high).*

By placing a copy of your own rules (boundaries) in a prominent position, they act as a reinforcing ritual when you read them daily.

Place them where you will read them as you rise in the morning. Try reading them out loud for an even greater impact!

Once your boundaries are set, you are ready for self-reflection – to evaluate the situation - when you find your boundaries slipping. The key is to stay **On Target** by remembering…

OK to slip up sometimes, as this is a learning process.

Nip the boundary slips in the bud as soon as possible.

Take each slipped boundary and deal with it separately.

Acknowledge the boundaries you are positively working within.

Remember to give yourself lots of positive feedback and praise.

Gather information on the triggers that create the boundary slips.

Execute action to overcome triggers and to prevent them happening again.

Techniques for 're-targeting' – build a list of ways to get back on track

'RE-TARGETING' TECHNIQUES
What do I mean by 'Re-targeting'? It is a way of refocusing yourself on your boundaries. Where you know you have a habit of overstepping a particular boundary it can be really useful. Knowing the triggers that cause your boundary to slips is the first step (e.g. stress, loneliness, emotional turmoil). Finding any actions you take that trigger the boundary slips can also be very useful (e.g. using the TV as a means of withdrawing from issues or emotions, which then leads to you eating inappropriately).

One of my triggers was coming home to an empty house. All my decisions about an evening of self-love and pampering would fly out of the window as soon as I crossed the threshold. Sometimes I could re-set the boundaries quickly. Most of the time the feeling of loneliness and isolation was too strong and I would withdraw from the world, my issue and just eat.

What was missing was someone to talk with, to share my day with. Most of all I missed someone to lift my spirits with some fun and laughter. That was a role my twin sister had always played. It was a role I never realised was available from deep within myself. All it took was a small funny looking bear called Spotty! Just seeing him makes me smile and releases my playful nature. So now he sits on a chair in my hall awaiting my attention and tales of the day, each time I come through the door.

Yes, it felt strange and funny to begin with, playing with a bear and talking to myself, but what did that matter when the results were so amazingly easy. Then something else happened. I began to pick him up, play and talk to him, as I decided what I wanted to eat or how to spend my time alone. Gone was the rebellion. Lost were my cravings and even more remarkable was how easy it was to serve myself portions half the size I had eaten before. And the by-product of all this silly behaviour was a wonderful flow of self-created joy flowing straight into my 'happiness reservoir'.

Once you have identified your triggers and actions, there are a number of ways that you can 'Re-target' yourself to overcome them...

- A repeated physical movement linked to a power statement e.g. a stroke of your hand when you feel yourself going into a stressful situation. This is then accompanied by a statement such as "This too will pass";
- A visual reminder (e.g. an easily accessible list of boundaries);
- A mental affirmation (i.e. a short sentence that you repeatedly chant in your mind);
- An action that becomes a ritual (e.g. a self-nurturing bath by candle light when the stress of life gets too much).

The choice is yours. What have you got to lose? Your happiness lies within the circle of your sound and well kept boundaries. Building a daily ritual of self-reflection and re-targeting is a major key to your success.

HONESTY IS THE BEST POLICY

Your ability to self-reflect and re-target is dependant on your level of self-honesty. When you are honest with yourself it builds a platform of authenticity. To be authentic is to hold true to your new beliefs, decisions and actions. This is the launch pad for your journey. Without being honest with yourself the launch pad will be built on an unstable platform, sabotaging your successful journey right from the beginning.

Even in the face of opposition, holding true to yourself enables you to regain your personal power, confidence and self-love. In the past it may have appeared easier to be economical with the truth, especially when faced with other people's judgment.

The more you focus on your journey towards happiness and your potential, the more you will be challenged to be honest and true to yourself. The aim of fear is to prevent you from attaining this level of honesty through its use of guilt and shame.

Be honest with yourself at least. Think how many times you have deceived yourself and others about what, and how much you eat. How much of your eating do you hide? How many times have you denied that you ate that last chocolate biscuit/cake/pudding? What a relief it will be for you, when you finally acknowledge that you have nothing to deny or hide.

With a mindset of 'Abundance' there really is nothing to feel ashamed or guilty of because there is no 'good' or 'bad' food thinking. Personal choice based on what makes you happy is the key. Linking this with 'Conscious Eating' and being in touch with your body and fuel tank signals, there really is no need to be anything other than honest. Acknowledge your overindulgence or inappropriate eating. Forgive yourself or others and get back on the track of your 'Abundant' mindset easily by being totally honest with yourself.

One of the ways that I would easily slip off track was through my inner rebellion of overeating. In childhood I had used food as a form of rebellion against what I saw as my father's overly controlling parenting. Part of it was a cry for attention. Inside I was screaming, "See me, love me and spend time with me."

Another part of the rebellion was taking control over something my father did not control – the food I ate. My rebellion was inappropriate and self-harming. In adulthood I found myself continuing these same habits with food. This time it was a rebellion against myself and remained so until I was honest enough to look at what my behaviour was trying to tell me.

On reflection, the realisation of what my rebellion was teaching me was amazing. When I was honest with myself and stopped blaming my father, I began to see that my rebellious overeating formed a repetitive pattern of behaviour. No longer was it a cry for attention from my father but from myself. It was my inner child crying out to be seen, listened to, loved and pampered by me! It always corresponded with times when I was too busy to allow myself any 'Me Time'. Getting back on track by giving myself the time and attention I needed to 'Feed My Soul', raising my energy and activity levels was the key.

Be honest with yourself about the foods that fill you with happiness and those that leave you, after a few minutes, feeling unhappy or really low. You know which ones I mean. They are not bad foods; they just don't make you happy and therefore are not self-loving. Don't forget that happiness is your birthright. It is up to you to make all the choices that draw it to you and keep it in your life.

Remember, you are only human and will make a choice every now and again that doesn't bring you happiness. When this happens there are two easy ways of dealing with it...

1. Admit to yourself that you really enjoyed whatever it was you ate, as you don't often have it. Savour the enjoyment of it. Remind yourself that it is always abundant and you can have it again whenever you want. Contrary to what you might think, you will not binge on it, as it is no longer scarce in your life.

OR

2. Focus on how unhappy the food or lack of activity made you feel and any negative physical effects it had on you. Exaggerate them in your mind. Use this as a reminder of how unhappy and uncomfortable the food or lack of activity made you feel. Use it to propel you back on track within your boundaries and rules.

Don't be frightened of food or honesty any more. It is fear that hinders your happiness. Keep true to yourself, your boundaries, your 'Nurturing Spirit' and choices for happiness.

LIVING LIFE TO THE 'MAX'

Another important part of honesty is recognising how much you focus on food, weight, size and shape. Living a life completely focused on these elements means that living life to the full is virtually impossible. It is your battle with food and life that makes happiness and living life to the full so illusive.

That is, if you have never met another of your inner friends, the Max. Decorated for his bravery in helping you face your demons, Max is the part of you which believes in the abundance of everything in life. He is the part of you that, if allowed, will

139

encourage you to stretch yourself to overcome your negative thoughts and fears in order to live life to the full.

Fearless in the extreme, yet empathetic and understanding of your barriers to change, Max knows the truth about your potential and the fears that holds you back from it. He knows they come from a belief in scarcity and not believing you are 'good enough'.

Max is the perfect friend for those seeking to find and live to their full potential. With a philosophy that life is not a rehearsal, Max makes sure that every possible opportunity to learn, have fun and enjoy life is taken.

If you allow him to, he will tell you all the positive reasons why you can do the things you have always shied away from. He will challenge your negative, scarcity thoughts and beliefs. He will encourage you, all the time, to love and accept yourself no matter what your size and shape.

Living life to 'The Max' meant finding and trusting myself, whilst gradually seeing the abundance in everything around me. Following a lifetime of believing only negative things about myself, it took courageous steps to move me towards finding my personal potential. For my first challenge, Max suggested I fulfil a life long dream to do a scuba dive on Australia's, Great Barrier Reef. Was he out of his mind! I was over 21 stone (a size 30), would have to be squeezed into an aircraft seat and need a miracle to get a wet suit on, let alone off.

"It may be your only chance." "Don't pass it by." "Just think what you will see." "So who cares what others may think." "There will be those who see your courage and determination." "Just think of how elated you will feel when you have done it", Max whispered encouragingly to me, when I was prepared to listen.

His persistence and patience finally paid off. Although it took three attempts to overcome the fear and get me down amongst the fish and coral, it was an experience of a lifetime. That was the first fear I overcame. Nothing could have prepared me for the way my courage and confidence grew, or the life that was opening up to me. After that, Max became my life long companion. I gained the confidence to travel alone to distant places. I developed closer friendships, placing the fear of rejection to one side. My courage knew no bounds, as I found more confidence to live life to the full.

So how can you start living your life to the 'MAX' now?

LIVING IN JOY

This is different from any weight loss journey you have been on before. It doesn't depend on listening to people telling you what to do, what to eat, how you should look or what foods are 'bad' or 'good'. All the decisions are up to you, so there is no need to deceive yourself or others, or hold back from life because of fear. "Yes, I did eat some chocolate and I really enjoyed it!" or "Yes, I will overcome my fear of heights by doing that Giant Redwood treetop walk". That's the stance to take.

So it is time to live in the moment, without a focus on food. This is where the joy of living is to be found. Even in moments of great sadness there is always beauty and joy to be seen. The key is to focus on the present. Take the gift of joy that it contains and use it wisely, for within it love abides.

Resonate the love within you. Feel its flow and glow. Give it freely to yourself first and then to others. For joy is experienced as love flows to you in abundance. Accept whatever the moment brings to you. Learn from it, forgive within it, have fun with it, seek answers from it and most of all seek peace within it. With peace comes joy, with joy comes love and where love is there is always happiness. The comfort you find here is in love not food.

Love can perform miracles because it heals all problems and dispels fear. Fear is the fundamental basis of the 'Scarcity' mindset. This is why, when the steps on your journey to an 'Abundant' mindset are filled with joy and love, and not food and fear, the miracle of weight loss is permanent.

The fact is you are the miracle. When you live in the moment with self-love in your heart and joy in your mind, food really does become just a fuel for your body. It is then that your potential to find the weight you were born to be becomes the reality.

The Top 10 Tips

For Your Future Journey

1. Remember, this is your journey created from the actions that resonate for you.

2. Make sure some of the actions are daily ones.

3. Make sure the actions you choose fill you with motivation.

4. Keep your motivation high by changing your plans whenever you want.

5. Remember there is no right way only YOUR way.

6. Make sure the actions bring you joy and happiness.

7. Have fun when you take action.

8. Remember, this is a life-change NOT a 'quick fix', so enjoy the process.

9. Don't let others distract you from your journey.

10. Believe in the power of your own potential.

Actions To Find Your Potential

1 Feed Your Soul With…your **New Actions For Change!**
Any journey begins with a clear action plan. So it is time, if you want to begin your journey, to make new choices for change. This is your journey, not mine. Choose carefully from the ideas, keys and techniques that I have described. Find those actions that resonate with you and keep your plan simple. Include in your plan some actions from each of the following categories…

- Seeing the abundance in your life;
- Feeding your mind with positive thoughts and emotions;
- 'Feeding Your Soul' through self-loving actions;
- 'Conscious Eating' techniques;
- Mind and body connections;
- Increased physical activity;
- 'Me Time';
- Noticing and absorbing positive strokes from others;
- Honesty, authenticity and personal power;
- Gratefulness and happiness;
- The healing of forgiveness;
- Loving your body image
- Personal boundaries.

Make your plans achievable on a daily basis. When life gets tough consider making your plan a focus of strength to help you through. Remember, these are the times your plan can easily slip. They are also the times when you need more love and support. Don't withdraw love from yourself just when you need more of it. Most of all have fun loving life, living life and letting go of old habits or beliefs.

2 Journey Log

This is a time of reflection. Look back at your journal/scrapbook, if you have already started one, or reflect back over the pages of this book that have resonated with you. Write down the things that come to mind as you use your self-reflection process.

Celebrate the actions and successes you have already achieved. Finally, integrate, into your action plan for change, the things your 'TARGET' reflections highlights as important to you.

Enjoy your new journey, share it with others, support others and most of all love the pure uniqueness of who you truly are.

143

GLOSSARY

Abundant Mindset
A mindset where there is no fear of food. An enjoyment of the abundance of food, love, joy and happiness. Where mind, body and spirit work in harmony with food and nature. Where weight loss is permanent.

Bank of Me
Time that you allocate and set aside in which to spend 'Me Time'.

Belief Systems
Deeply held beliefs, both positive and negative that you develop in childhood, some of which may no longer be useful to you in adulthood (e.g. believing you're 'not good enough').

Body Image
How you currently view – love or hate – your body as it is in the present moment.

Comfort Eating
The intake of food when not hungry for fuel on which to run your body but when hungry for love, attention and emotional healing.

Conscious Eating
The ability to fully connect your mind to be in tune with your body and its needs, when you are eating, viewing and using food. The habits with food that people who have never dieted use.

Discounting
Throwing away positive 'strokes' / 'magic messages' because they are not heard, believed or valued by the recipient or because they make them feel uncomfortable.

Fat Jacket
Excess weight around you that has built up over many years of yo-yo dieting or inappropriate eating.

Feeding Your Soul
The loving actions you take each day that lift your spirits. The people, places and events that lift your spirits and make them soar with love and gratitude.

Good Enough
A high level of confidence, self-worth and self-belief where you do not judge yourself against others. Where you love yourself as you currently are, no matter what your shape, size and weight, but you still lose weight.

Happiness Fix
External communications, actions or events that bring happiness.

Inner Voice
The voice of your deep intuition that can guide you if you are willing to be still enough to listen.

Journey Log
A personal journal of your self-discovery that can motivate when used as a tool for self-reflective learning.

Not Good Enough
A belief that unless you are on a diet, losing weight or have achieved a certain shape, size or weight you are not acceptable to yourself or others.

Love Power
An ability to truly love yourself enough to look after your needs as if you were your own best friend.

Magic Messages
Positive 'strokes' of communication or action that can raise motivation, giving the recipient a glow of loving warmth, when the message is accepted and valued.

Me Time
Time that you spend on yourself doing things that nurture you and 'Feed Your Soul'.

Mind/Body Connection
Where your mind is actively switched onto the feelings of your body.

Motivation
A belief in yourself and your ability to achieve your goals, inspired by seeing and believing the positive, loving things within and around you.

Nurturing Spirit
A loving energy around and within you, in all living things, that has only your best interest at heart and that you can tap into to 'Feed Your Soul'.

Perfect Selfishness
The right to be selfish with some of your time and spend it doing things that are self-loving and 'Feed Your Soul'.

Personal Power
The undertaking of positive actions based on self-choice, where you stand up for what you believe is right for you and where you are not influenced by others to go against your values, boundaries and decisions.

Pit of Despair
A place of frustration and unhappiness experienced when yo-yo dieting and when shame, guilt and self-loathing are prevalent.

Scarcity Mindset
The mindset of a dieter where life is a battle with food and self-belief. Where there is a belief in 'good'/'bad' food, weight loss is a destination and food is feared. Where there is a belief that you are 'Not Good Enough' unless you are a certain shape, size and weight.

The Body's Set Point
The weight, size & shape your body was born to be.

The Max
That part of you that challenges and encourages you to stretch yourself to realise your full potential and live life to the full

The Pro
Procrastination; that part within you which encourages you to give up on positive action and do it another time, giving you all the excuses you need to justify your non-action.

What Is
Things in your life that are certain and that you have no power to change (e.g. short legs like your mother)

ABOUT THE AUTHOR

Chrissie Webber works as a writer, coach and leadership trainer. She is also Managing Director of Life Shapers Ltd, an online motivational weight management company. An experienced presenter and public speaker, Chrissie has a passion for helping people stretch themselves to reach their full potential and find the weight they were born to be.

Following a lifetime of weight issues - at her heaviest, over 21 stone and a massive size 30 – she has personal experience of diets and their devastating effect on size and psyche. Her background in nursing and psychology enabled her to successfully develop and use a series of models and tools that enhance weight loss motivation. Now over 5 dress sizes smaller, having sustained her weight loss for several years, Chrissie continues her passionate drive to change people's demotivating, dieting mindsets.

Her work continues, establishing a team of Weight Loss Motivation Coaches offering a network of local support groups. She also has a web site at *www.lifeshapers.co.uk* providing a range of motivational services including a Daily Weight Loss Motivation Programme and a free monthly ezine. Her Blog *www.chrissiewebber.co.uk* offers motivational support and an opportunity for others to discuss the issues with her.

Chrissie lives in South Wales and has two married daughters.